To
Gregg,
Be good to your body!

BODY-LIFE NOW!

Mini-Meditations for Maximum Fitness Motivation

BODY-LIFE NOW!

Mini-Meditations for Maximum Fitness Motivation

by

Bishop Jim Earl Swilley

Body-Life Now!
Mini-Meditations for Maximum Fitness Motivation
ISBN 0-9716838-3-2
Copyright ©2004 by Jim Earl Swilley

1st Printing: 2004
Printer: United Book Press, Inc., Baltimore, MD
Cover designer: Chris Haler, Current Events Productions, Covington, GA
Bio photograph: Chris & Teri Haler, Current Events Productions, Covington, GA
Technical/Production Editors: René Babcock, Jane Conyers, Robyn Darby

Published by Church In The Now Publishing
1873 Iris Drive, SE
Conyers, GA 30013

CONTENTS

BODY-LIFE NOW!

INTRODUCTION

Mini-Meditations* for Maximum** Fitness Motivation***

*Meditate: *1. Engage in deep thought; reflect. 2. Plan mentally (think, ponder, study, ruminate, cogitate, contemplate, cerebrate).*

Total fitness flows from the inside out. The physical aspect is only one part of it. Meditation improves *spiritual* and *mental* fitness, and allows the physical to become a manifestation of inner health and strength.

**Maximum: *Highest possible or attainable amount (utmost, uttermost, greatest, most, highest, extreme, limit, peak, pinnacle).*

Total fitness is absolutely attainable, and the work that must be done to achieve it is definitely doable. Anyone who deeply desires to realize their whole potential can certainly do so.

***Motivate: *1. Supply a motive to; be the motive of. 2. Stimulate the interest of (prompt, activate, move, inspire, incite, excite).*

Total fitness requires constant motivation . . .
motivation to *get* fit . . .
motivation to *stay* fit.

Motivation is necessary for the whole person . . .
spirit, soul and body.

Invigorate my soul so I can praise you well, use your decrees to put iron in my soul. (Psalm 119:175)

1.   PRIORITIES

. . . Exercise daily in God – no spiritual flabbiness, please! Workouts in the gymnasium are useful, but a disciplined life in God is far more so, making you fit both today and forever. (1 Timothy 4:7,8)

In your workout today, remember that the *spiritual* always comes before the *physical.*

The spiritual is *eternal*; the physical is *temporal.*

You are not a *natural* person trying to gain access to the spiritual realm;

You are a *spiritual* person manifesting yourself in the material world.

You *are* a **spirit**.

You *have* a **soul**.

You *live* in a **body**.

But that doesn't mean that the physical is not important.

Without a physical body, you would have no authority on this planet.

Your body is an exquisite gift from God to you, and should be cared for, appreciated, and honored.

God's first commandment was for man to subdue the earth and take dominion over it,

and the human body was created from the dust of that earth.

So when you discipline *yours* to make it better, stronger, leaner, harder,

you are subduing a part of the *earth* and taking dominion over it.

God looked at His finished creation and said, "It is *good.*"

He did not say that it was *perfect.*

He placed man in the garden and gave him orders to take the good earth that He had created,

and cultivate and *improve* it, because He wanted man to be involved in the creative process.

When you take the body that God gave you to a higher level of excellence,

when you maximize its potential, you are doing a good thing–a Kingdom thing.

But, remember that the spiritual *always* comes first.

BODY-LIFE NOW!

2. PURPOSE

. . . The physical part of you is not some piece of property belonging to the spiritual part of you. God owns the whole works. So let people see God in and through your body. (1 Corinthians 6:19,20)

———————

The purpose of exercise is to glorify God in your body.

The purpose of weight training is to glorify God in your body.

The purpose of walking, running, or doing any other cardiovascular-improving activity

is to glorify God in your body.

The purpose of aerobics, calisthenics, stretching –

any pursuit that develops muscular tone,

or promotes physical well-being –

is good, positive – even godly.

Your body is a temple–a sacred place.

Every beneficial physical activity should be engaged in with a certain *reverence* for the sacred.

God is holy, and you are created in His image and likeness.

So lift, push, pull, move, bend, stretch, and build as an act of *worship* –

a giving of thanks to the Creator for the marvelous works of His hand.

Breathe deeply, knowing that every breath is a gift from Him.

Your blood is pumping.

Your heart is beating.

Your body is perspiring.

You are alive!

Even the pain is a reminder that you are *alive* and *feeling* and *growing* and *changing*!

Your life has purpose.

To God be the glory!

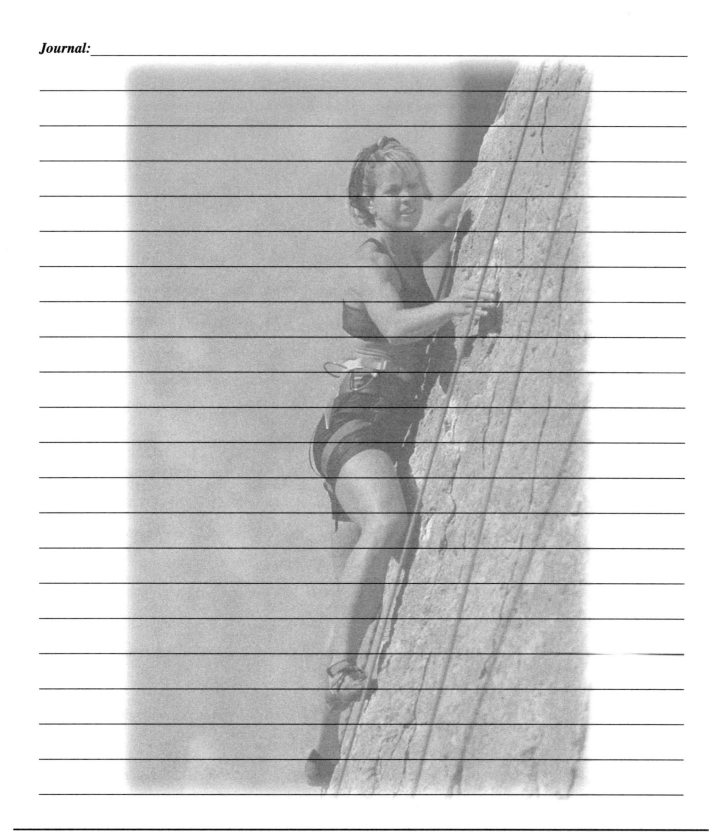

3. MOTIVATION

God answer you on the day you crash . . . give you what your heart desires, accomplish your plans. When you win, we plan to raise the roof and lead the parade with our banners. May all your wishes come true! (Psalm 20:1,4,5)

—————◆—————

Yes, you can! Yes, you will! Yes, you should! Yes, you must!

You are strong! You are able! You are disciplined! You are committed!

You are a fighter! You are a trooper! You are a champion! You are a winner!

You have the power! You have the stamina! You have the opportunity! You have the will!

Your time is now! Your season is now! Your day is today! Your victory is here!

You can't quit now! You can't give up! You can't give in! You can't lose out!

You've got to be determined and diligent! You've got to be aggressive and strong!

You need to get up! You need to get going! You need to get busy! You need to get moving!

You must have a goal and a plan! You must hold on to your dream and stay true to your vision!

You've got to believe and keep trying! You've got to keep working and push yourself!

You're *not* going to fail or lose! You're *not* going to be disappointed or be "less than!"

You are worth the effort! You are worth the investment! You are valuable! You are *somebody*!

You're not too *old!* You're not too *weak!* You're not too *fat!* You're not too *lazy!*

You *know* how to do it and that you have it in you! You *know* you want to and that you can!

You have the potential! You have the desire! You have the mindset! You have the time!

You don't have to make excuses or be mediocre! You don't have to settle or put it off!

You're going to achieve your goals and go to the next level! You're going to make it and excel!

You can stand the pain! You can overcome the obstacles! You can get stronger! You can do better!

You've got to keep going! You've got to keep the promise you made to yourself and keep trying!

You have what it takes! You have the edge! You have the attitude! You have the energy!

God is good! God is great! God is for you! God is helping you today!

Journal: _____

_____

_____

_____

_____

_____

_____

_____

BODY-LIFE NOW!

_____

_____

_____

_____

_____

_____

_____

4. STRENGTH

I'm feeling terrible – I couldn't feel worse! Get me on my feet again. You promised, remember? When I told my story, you responded; train me well in your deep wisdom. Help me understand these things inside and out so I can ponder your miracle-wonders. My sad life's dilapidated, a falling-down barn; build me up again by your Word. (Psalm 119:25-28)

You can build up and strengthen your inner self by the Word of God

in the same way that you build up your physical body by working out with weights.

Claim these seven promises for *yourself* today –

– for everything that you are trying to accomplish in and around you

– for your workout, game or exercise

– for your spirit

– for your soul

– for your body.

You will find that you are stronger than you think you are.

The promises of God are *yes* and *amen*:

(1) *You are **strong** in the Lord, and in the power of His might! (Ephesians 6:10)*

(2) *You are **strengthened** with might, by His Spirit, in the inner man! (Ephesians 3:16)*

(3) *The joy of the Lord is your **strength**! (Nehemiah 8:10)*

(4) *Let the weak say I am **strong**! (Joel 3:10)*

(5) *The Lord is the **strength** of your life! (Psalm 27:1)*

(6) *You can do all things through Christ Who **strengthens** you! (Philippians 4:13)*

(7) *In your weakness, He is made **strong**! (2 Corinthians 12:9,10)*

You are getting stronger today and every day.

There is a greater, stronger, more powerful *you* on the inside that is trying to come out.

You can release him/her by meditating the Word of God and believing it – mixing it with faith.

Be strong today. Be the best you can be. Do everything to the glory of God.

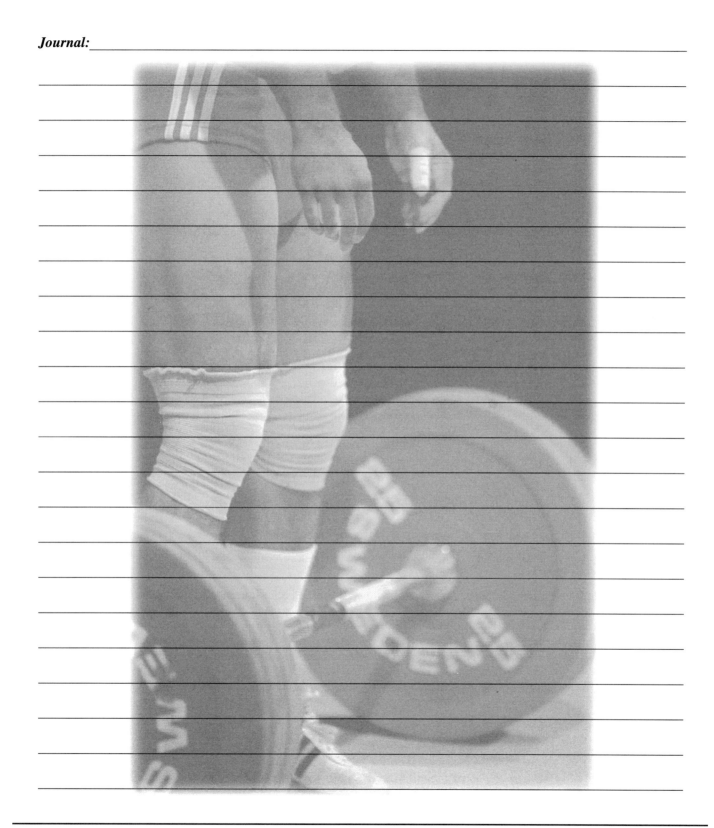

5. DISCIPLINE

At the time, DISCIPLINE isn't much fun. It always feels like it's going against the grain. Later, of course, it pays off handsomely, for it's the well-trained who find themselves mature in their relationship with God. (Hebrews 12:11)

———•••———

The Scripture says: *"Where there is no vision the people perish."*

It is better translated from the Hebrew language:
"Where there is no revelation (prophetic vision) the people cast off restraint."

A vision enables you to stay disciplined.

It keeps you from "casting off restraint."

It motivates you to get up in the morning and start working toward your goal.

Vision is a vivid, inner picture of a future reality.

Discipline without vision is drudgery and will inevitably cause burnout.

But vision-driven discipline is a *lifestyle*.

It's the lifestyle of a winner.

It's the lifestyle of a champion.

It's a lifestyle that pays off at the end of the day.

You must have an inner picture of how you want to be (to look - to feel) on the outside.

The picture must be *realistic* and *achievable*,

but it should be *big* enough, *challenging* enough, and *desirable* enough to make you want to work for it.

Discipline is preparation. Discipline is training.

Discipline is a habit. Discipline is the way to greatness.

Discipline separates the men from the boys, the women from the girls.

Discipline brings the inner picture into focus, day by day.

Discipline is being willing to work hard *today* for the reward *tomorrow*.

Discipline is maintaining the ability to see what others can't see,

and protecting and preserving that vision at all times.

*Journal:*_____

_____

_____

_____

_____

_____

_____

BODY-LIFE NOW!

_____

_____

_____

_____

_____

_____

_____

_____

_____

_____

6. POWER

And that about wraps it up. God is strong, and he wants you strong. (Ephesians 6:10)

———◦—◦———

God has given you the power to do something positive with your life.

You have the power to realize your destiny –

to take what He has given you and make it the best that it can be.

Who you *are* is God's gift to you.

Who you *become* is your gift to God.

Working out or exercising should be just *one part* of the overall plan to maximize your potential.

It's not the only thing.

It's not even the most important thing.

You are much more than your physical body.

You have the power to do good.

You have the power to inspire others.

You have the power to help somebody.

You have the power to make the world around you a better place.

Strengthen your arms so that you can use them to build bridges and tear down walls.

Strengthen your legs so that you can run with your vision for a better tomorrow.

Strengthen your shoulders so that you can carry more responsibility in your community.

Strengthen your back so that you can help someone else bear their burden.

Strengthen your chest so that it will be big enough for others to lean on.

Celebrate the reality that you have been empowered to control your own destiny . . .

to do good.

You've got the *power!*

Journal:

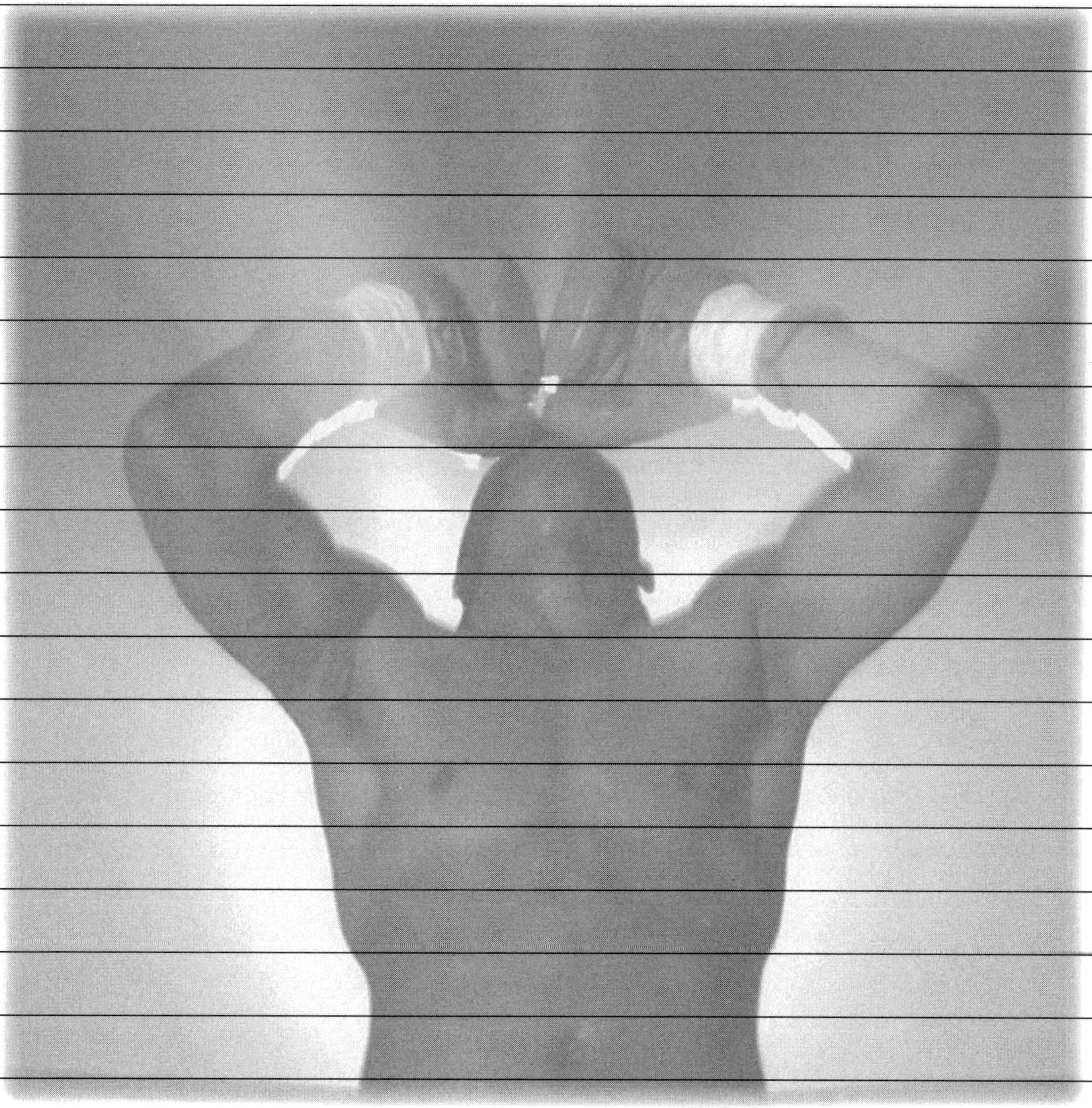

7. HEALTH

. . . I pray for good fortune in everything you do, and for your GOOD HEALTH – that your everyday affairs prosper, as well as your soul! (3 John 2)

—————

God created man to be *healthy*.

God created man to be *whole*.

A healthy body is the product of a healthy mind.

A healthy *mind* manifests a healthy *attitude*, which promotes a healthy *lifestyle*.

Healthy thoughts create healthy words:

*. . . there is **healing** in the words of the wise. (Proverbs 12:18)*

*Kind words **heal** and help . . . . (Proverbs 15:4)*

Words satisfy the mind as much as fruit does the stomach;

good talk is as gratifying as a good harvest.

Words kill, words give life; they're either poison or fruit – you choose. (Proverbs 18:20,21)

***Thoughts** become **words**. Words become **deeds**.*

Deeds become ***habits***. Habits become ***lifestyle***.

Lifestyle becomes ***character***. Character becomes ***destiny***.

It is important to eat right, to breathe deeply, to get enough rest, and to drink plenty of water.

But it is *counterproductive* to try to maintain a healthy body while your *mind* is full of negativity

and your *heart* is full of bitterness, hatred, doubt, and unbelief.

The definition of disease is "dis-ease" –

the *dis-ease* of spirit, soul, and body.

You must become healthy from the inside out.

When that happens, you will not just be healthy –

you will be *whole*.

*Journal:*_____

BODY-LIFE NOW!

8.   MOVEMENT

We live and MOVE in him, can't get away from him! One of your poets said it well: "We're the God-created."
(Acts 17:28)

————•—•————

Movement is not just about increasing heart rate.

It's not just about boosting metabolism or burning calories and fat.

It's about *celebrating* the energy of life!

It's about gracefulness, balance, flexibility, flow of motion –

– the awareness of the life-force

– the ability to tap into unknown sources of strength

– the miracle of the second-wind.

Movement is about not being stuck in one place

and, therefore, it has great symbolism for your life.

It represents change, and change is good.

You are not stuck!

You are in *motion* . . . in *transition* . . . in the *flow*.

Ultimately, movement is about uninhibited praise:

Then David danced before the Lord WITH ALL HIS MIGHT . . . . (2 Samuel 6:14)

All of God's creation is in motion.

The earth is revolving and rotating on its axis.

The wind is blowing; the grass is growing.

Scientists have proven that even the rocks are moving.

When you move today, you are joining with all of nature

to participate in one cosmic dance.

Let everything that has breath praise the Lord!

---

*Journal:*_____

_____

_____

_____

_____

_____

_____

_____

_____

_____

_____

_____

_____

_____

_____

_____

9. STAMINA

Suddenly, God, you floodlight my life; I'm blazing with glory, God's glory! I smash the bands of marauders, I vault the highest fences. (Psalm 18:28,29)

———————

Stamina is strength, endurance, the ability to keep up the pace –

– to get back up when you fall

– to step up to the plate when you don't feel like it

– to run and not be weary

– to walk and not faint.

For your workout or exercise, stamina is important

and is helped by vitamins, nutrition, and a positive attitude.

For your *life*, stamina is even more important.

If you fall to pieces in a crisis,

there wasn't much to you in the first place. (Proverbs 24:10)

You have a purpose.

You have a destiny.

God has a plan for your life.

There was a reason for your birth.

You have a reason to live.

You have a reason to keep going.

Think of all the things that you've already survived, and realize that

that which did not kill you only served to make you *stronger*.

In your physical workouts, you've made too much progress to quit now.

In your *life*, you've come too far to turn back.

The only way out is *through*. The only direction allowed is *forward*.

BODY-LIFE NOW!

10. BODY

Oh yes, you shaped me first inside, then out; you formed me in my mother's womb. I thank you, High God – you're breathtaking! BODY and soul, I am marvelously made! I worship in adoration – what a creation! You know me inside and out, you know every bone in my BODY; you know exactly how I was made, bit by bit, how I was sculpted from nothing into something. (Psalm 139:13-15)

———◆———

You were made in God's likeness.

You were created in His image.

Your eyes were made to see the revelation of the brightness of His glory.

Your ears were made to hear the thunder of His mighty voice.

Your hands were made to creatively help your fellow man.

Your arms were made to reach up to heaven in praise and worship.

Your feet were made to follow in His footsteps.

Your body is His temple.

You were born to be His dwelling place – a home for His presence.

Your own "temple" is a mechanism of miracles –

a walking testimonial to the existence of the living God.

It's made out of good stuff, so you can push it to the extreme.

You can work it hard, knowing that its high quality will be self-sustaining.

The handiwork of God is seen in your entire body –

– in your muscles, tendons, sinews, joints, and ligaments

– in your limbs, and the bones that support them

– in your fingers and toes

– in your internal organs.

The human body is a beautiful, amazing thing.

It is one of God's crowning achievements.

When you exercise yours today, treat it like the *masterpiece* that it is!

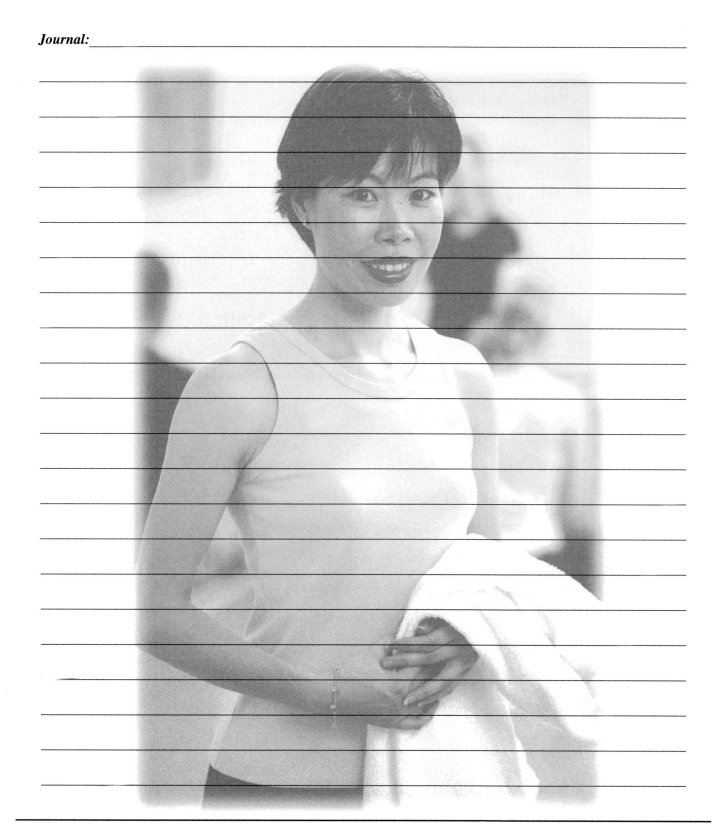

11. WALKING

But those who wait upon God get fresh strength. They spread their wings and soar like eagles, They run and don't get tired, they WALK and don't lag behind. (Isaiah 40:31)

———◆◆———

Walking is good for your *heart* and good for your *head*.

Whether inside on the treadmill – elevating your heart rate, breaking a sweat –

or outside in the beauty of God's awesome creation – breathing deeply, feeling the sunshine on your skin;

whether early in the morning, as you develop the attitude and vision for your day –

or at sunset, as you wind down, thanking God for bringing you successfully through another one –

keep walking, no matter what. You must face forward and *move*.

Step by step, you are advancing toward better health of body and mind.

Step by step, you are moving into a whole new dimension.

Today is your day to pick up the pace and *keep* it up.

Feel the power in your legs – your thighs, your calves –

and know that you are doing something really good for yourself.

Timing is everything, and there is always time for better health.

Breathe a prayer while you stride along,

because the *inner* man is keeping pace with the *outer* man in your walk.

Let the constant movement clear your head

and awaken your senses.

Maximize every quiet moment of your walk, because the day might be hectic and chaotic,

and this may be your only little window of opportunity to breathe, focus, and be at peace.

From casual strolling to intense power-walking – it's *all* good.

Keep going – there's no turning back.

And remember, today, that you are walking with God!

*Journal:*_____

_____

_____

_____

_____

_____

_____

_____

_____

BODY-LIFE NOW!

_____

_____

_____

_____

_____

_____

_____

_____

12. RUNNING

Is there any god like God? Are we not at bedrock? Is not this the God who armed me, then aimed me in the right direction? Now I RUN like a deer; I'm king of the mountain. (Psalm 18:31-33)

—◆—

You have responded to your innate need for speed.

With the wind in your face, you begin to feel like you could run forever;

the movement activates a feeling from deep within that all things really *are* possible.

Running, jogging, sprinting . . .

competitive running, or just doing it for your own well-being . . .

it just feels right.

You're not just burning calories . . . you begin to feel that you're burning bridges behind you.

Your heart rate keeps you aware that you are living in the *now*.

Everything is moving in sync . . .

legs, arms, feet, ankles, knees, toes, shins, thighs, calves . . .

bones, muscles, joints and tendons are in harmony.

The stress is relieved.

The pressure is put into perspective.

Your eyes become more focused.

The intake of oxygen to your brain heightens your awareness of the world around you

as the rhythm of your heartbeat accelerates.

Run on.

Run with your vision.

Run, and do not be weary.

Run like the champion that you are.

Run for your *life*!

*Journal:*_____

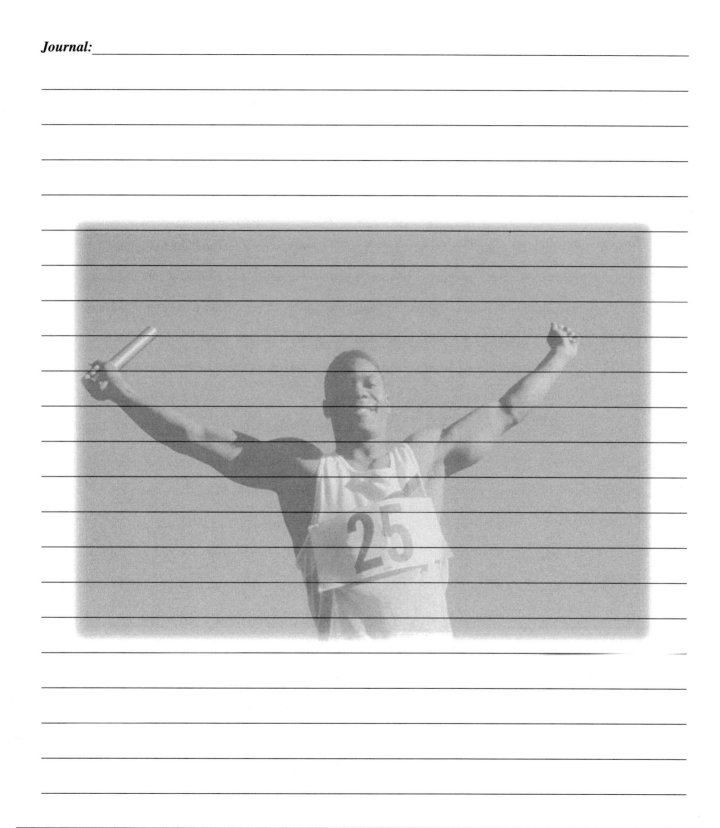

13.   SELF-ESTEEM

God will make you the head, not the tail; you'll always be top dog, never the bottom dog, as you obediently listen to and diligently keep the commands of God, your God, that I am commanding you today.
(Deuteronomy 28:13)

———◆———

The great commandment is to love God with all of your heart,

and to love your neighbor as you love *yourself*.

The question, then, is this: How can you love another until you have learned to love yourself?

How can you expect another to believe in you, if you don't believe in yourself?

You are not perfect, but you *are* valuable, important and worthy of respect – including *self*-respect.

Properly balanced self-love empowers you to be good to yourself and to nurture your whole being.

Speaking positive words about yourself enables you to believe that
it is *commendable* and *admirable* to take care of your body.

You are neither superior nor inferior to anyone else. You are unique!

Some might say that caring about the quality and appearance of your physique is a sign of shallowness or pride –

that it's motivated by an over-inflated ego.

That's something that you will have to judge for yourself, because no one, except God,
can truly know your motives for doing

anything.

In his first letter to the church at Corinth, the Apostle Paul said that people could give all of their goods to feed the poor,

and even allow themselves to be martyred, all for wrong motives. He said that it would profit them nothing.

So, no one is qualified to judge *any* of your motives in *any* matter.

Besides, God doesn't want or need to destroy your ego,

He just wants you to submit it to His will.

So, if building your body builds your self-confidence and self-esteem,

it's not going to make God fall off His throne!

He is not intimidated by you, so go ahead and be the *best* that you can be.

*Journal:*_____

BODY-LIFE NOW!

14. MUSCLES

Fine MUSCLES ripple beneath his skin, quiet and beautiful. His torso is the work of a sculptor, hard and smooth as ivory. He stands tall, like a cedar, strong and deep-rooted, a rugged mountain of a man, aromatic with wood and stone. (Song of Solomon 5:14,15)

———◆———

Feel the strength of your muscles responding positively to the tension and the pressure.

You are growing and increasing as you push the weights and pull the weights, day after day.

Resistance makes you stronger as you repeatedly press the weight away from your body.

Little surprise bursts of energy motivate you to do one more set – to add a little *more* weight.

The power is intoxicating. You want to do it again. You want to come back for more tomorrow.

The vigor of your youth is awakened from its slumber as the blood races through your veins.

The force is with you as you find the perfect rhythm for your lifting and pumping. You are in the zone.

You feel the tone of your muscles improving – even the skin around them glows with the elasticity of life.

As you gradually begin to notice definition in different areas of your body, you see the emergence of

a whole new you that has been hiding – buried beneath the skin. You feel flexible, balanced and strong.

You've worked hard. Don't feel embarrassed to look in the mirror and admire the fruits of your labor.

Just say "thank you" when someone notices and comments in the affirmative. You *should* feel proud of your results.

God is not reluctant to show *His* might:

. . . He rolled up his sleeves, He set things right.

God made history with salvation, He showed the world what He could do. (Psalm 98:1,2)

He is not ashamed to show His *muscle*:

God has rolled up his sleeves.

All the nations can see his holy MUSCLED arm.

Everyone, from one end of the earth to the other,

sees him at work, doing his salvation work. (Isaiah 52:10)

Be strong in the Lord and in the power of His might!

Journal:

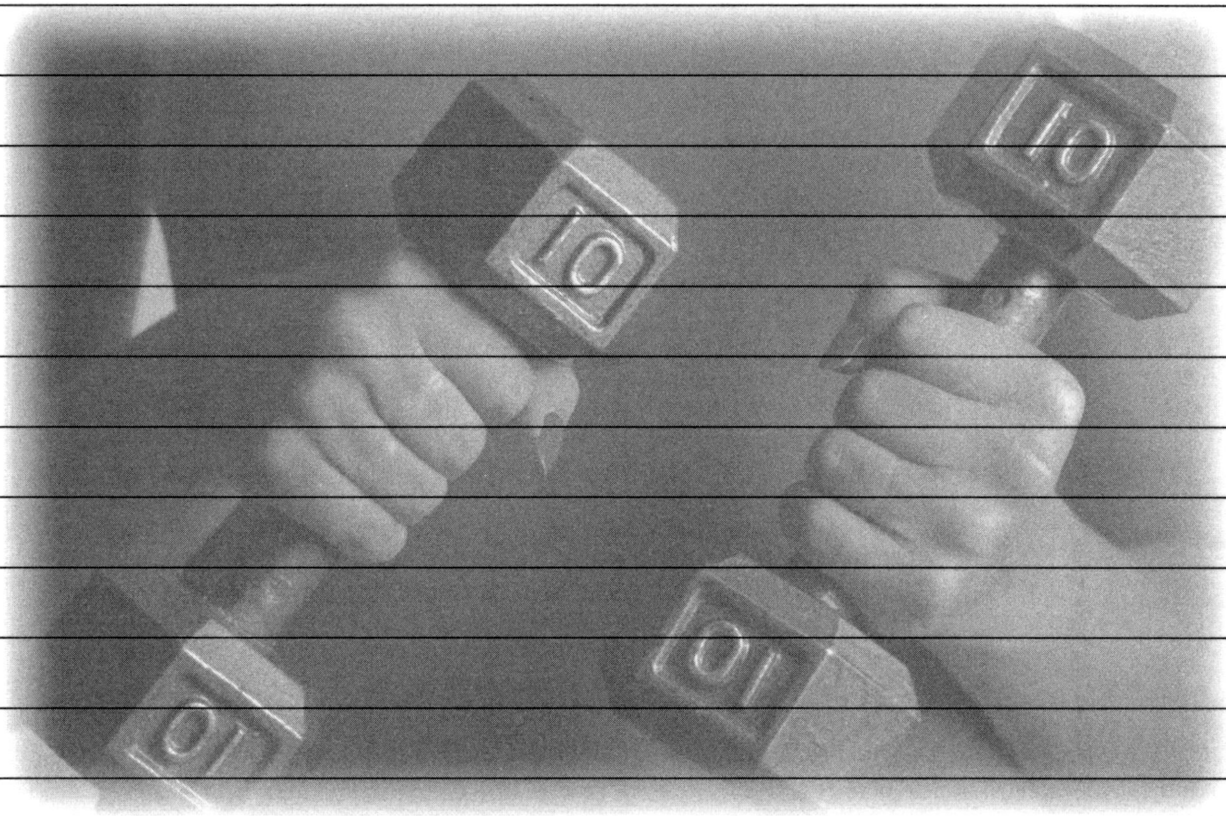

15. VISION

And then God answered: "Write this. Write what you see. Write it out in big block letters so that it can be read on the run. The VISION-message is a witness pointing to what's coming. It aches for the coming – it can hardly wait! And it doesn't lie. If it seems slow in coming, wait. It's on its way. It will come right on time." (Habakkuk 2:2,3)

—————

If you can see it, you can have it.

If you can believe it, you can achieve it.

. . . your old men shall dream dreams, your young men shall see visions. (Joel 2:28)

Vision perpetuates youth and vigor and faith and hope.

Don't just settle for developing an internal picture of what you want to *look* like;

embrace a *larger* picture of what you want to *be* like.

You are not just a human being . . .

you are a human *becoming*!

You are becoming something greater than you are right now.

For as he thinks in his heart, so is *he . . . .* (Proverbs 23:7)

Open wide the eyes of your heart,

and observe the vision birthed in your spirit.

Your body will conform to your inner man.

Fill up your words with your vision,

for your future is in your mouth.

You are a product today of what you said yesterday.

Tomorrow you will be what you are saying today.

But you can't *say* it if you can't *see* it.

Look ahead, because something good is coming.

Try to observe the appearance of the *you* that is on the way.

Look and live!

*Journal:*_____

BODY-LIFE NOW!

16.   YOUTHFULNESS

He wraps you in goodness – beauty eternal. He renews your YOUTH – you're always YOUNG in his presence.
(Psalm 103:5)

———◆·◆———

Exercise and muscle conditioning help to slow down, and even reverse, the human aging process.

Being physically fit makes you *feel* younger and *look* younger, and that alone is a great incentive for working out.

Jesus said that you must become child-like to enter the Kingdom

and, even though He was speaking of spiritual matters,

it *is* important to maintain a playful innocence and sense of wonder in *everything* that you do,

both spiritually and physically.

Today, let the kid in you find the *fun* again in your workout or exercise.

Discipline is crucial – but so is a sense of play –

so don't take it all so seriously.

Change your attitude and *enjoy* it once more.

Exercise *should* be a stress-reliever,

so decide to get the most out of it by letting the stress go.

Stress ages you and is counterproductive to your physical training.

Lighten up, already!

Laugh a little.

Begin each new day with a sense of adventure.

Make the most of life's little pleasures that you usually take for granted.

There is still a lot to be excited about in your life,

so let your pursuit of fitness help you to rediscover the joy of living.

God restores your youth like the eagle's.

And, remember, you're not getting *older*, you're getting *better!*

Journal:

17.   TRAINING

. . . Strip down, start running – and never quit! No extra spiritual fat, no parasitic sins. Keep your eyes on **Jesus,** *who both began and finished this race we're in. Study how he did it. Because he never lost sight of where he was headed – that exhilarating finish in and with God – he could put up with anything along the way: cross, shame, whatever. And now he's* **there,** *in the place of honor, right alongside God. When you find yourselves flagging in your faith, go over that story again, item by item, that long litany of hostility he plowed through.* **That** *will shoot adrenaline into your souls! (Hebrews 12:1-3)*

If it was easy, everybody would be doing it.

Discipline is worth it. It always pays off, eventually.

Your self-respect demands excellence of you, and so you train today, whether you feel like it or not.

The will to win is meaningless without the will to prepare,

so stop procrastinating, and do what you need to do.

Don't say that you don't have the time – you must *make* the time.

Today you are managing your life by bringing your body into order.

Today you are making your goals less abstract and shortening the distance between them and you.

Today you're getting a little bit stronger.

Today you're getting a little bit leaner.

Today your muscles are getting a little bit harder,

a little bit better defined.

Today you're going to feel a little bit better about yourself.

Today you're going to like what you see in the mirror a little bit more.

You can train your attitude,

so that you can more effectively train your body.

You can look forward to tomorrow, because tomorrow it starts all over again.

It is a continuous commitment – get used to it.

Your future is hidden in your daily routine.

Don't you dare be discouraged!

You can do it!

---

*Journal:*_____

_____

_____

_____

_____

_____

_____

BODY-LIFE NOW!

_____

_____

_____

_____

_____

_____

_____

18. BALANCE

It is better to be wise than strong; intelligence outranks muscle any day. (Proverbs 24:5)

———•◦•———

Balance is not just about body symmetry.

It is about the harmony of the spiritual with the physical.

Balance is being faithful to do something good for your spirit *and* mind *and* body every day.

Remember, even your workout is not just about the physical.

It's about clearing your mind so that it can be more productive,

and caring for the temple that houses your spirit.

The earth continuously revolves and gives us night and day, day and night.

The seasons are balanced – winter, spring, summer, fall . . .

light and dark . . .

hot and cold.

Everything in God's creation is balanced. Everything gives and everything takes.

To everything there is a season . . .

There is an important balance that you need between work and rest.

Be as disciplined in one as in the other.

When your body cries out for rest, it is really crying out for *balance*.

Take a day off every now and then from your regular routine.

Relax.

Get renewed and refreshed.

You can get back on schedule tomorrow.

It's *all* good!

It's all about the balance.

*Journal:*_____

19. TENACITY

When the going gets rough, take it on the chin with the rest of us, the way Jesus did. A soldier on duty doesn't get caught up in making deals in the marketplace. He concentrates on carrying out orders. An athlete who refuses to play by the rules will never get anywhere. It's the diligent farmer who gets the produce.
(2 Timothy 2:3-6)

———◆———

Don't give up!

Don't stop until you get *yours*!

Don't surrender anything.

Find the most stubborn part of your will and tap into it.

Go way down deep inside of yourself and dredge up all the strength that you can muster.

Get tough – get *mean* if you have to! You've got a job to do that *only you* can do.

Resist any temptation to be too easy on yourself. You are a champion, and you can take the pressure.

Resolve within yourself that quitting is not an option.

When you feel like you're at your breaking point, remember that you are the closest to your breakthrough,

so, laugh in the face of weakness – it is *not* your master.

Never say die. Never throw in the towel.

As cliché as it may be, you know it's true: No pain, no gain!

Get a tight grip on what you want to achieve and refuse to let go.

By your sheer will you are able to continue long after those who started with you have dropped out.

By your outstanding commitment, you prove that you are not like them.

You show up when they flake out, and it doesn't even slow you down.

You never thought it could happen, but now you actually *love* the discipline.

In your heart of hearts you truly believe that the world is full of possibilities,

and so you bounce back after having a bad day.

What happened yesterday is *nothing* in the grand scheme of things.

Ah, the power of the made-up mind!

*Journal:*_____

BODY-LIFE NOW!

20. CONCENTRATION

Your eyes are windows into your body. If you open your eyes wide in wonder and belief, your body fills up with light. (Matthew 6:22)

———

Keep your eyes on the prize.

When you're working out, really *concentrate* on what you are doing

and why you are doing it.

Be there *mentally*, as well as physically.

Put every distraction out of your mind.

Forget about who said what, or what you need to do later today.

This is *your* time. Use it wisely.

Harness your stress and recondition it into strength for your regimen.

Make it all work for your good.

Pay attention to your body and what it is saying to you right now.

Focus on the big picture.

Your body has been very faithful and consistent in its service to you

and, therefore, it deserves your undivided attention today.

Forget every negative thing that you're dealing with. It doesn't matter right now.

Imagine yourself well and strong and at peace with your environment.

Visualize your spirit, soul, and body being in perfect harmony.

Your mind is clear and decisive. You know the direction that you need to follow today.

The *real* you is awakening from its sluggish idleness.

You are peaceful, without being passive – calm, but not complacent.

Your dedication will pay off in due season.

Discover all the possibilities that are stored in the hidden rooms of your heart.

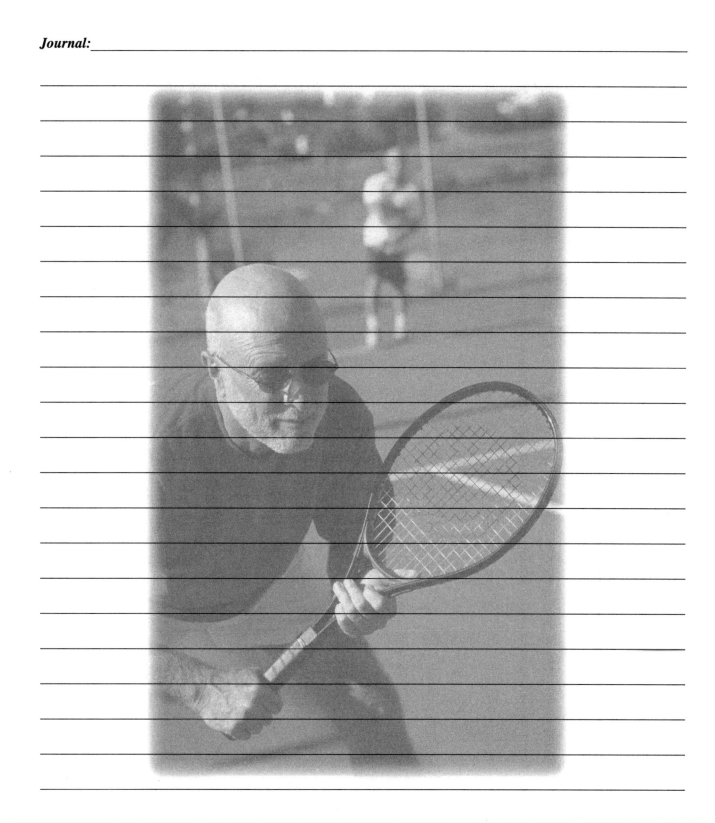

21. HABITS

The road to life is a disciplined life; ignore correction and you're lost for good. (Proverbs 10:17)

———◆———

1. Anything done consistently for 21 days becomes a habit.

2. Anything done consistently for 21 days becomes a habit.

3. Anything done consistently for 21 days becomes a habit.

4. Anything done consistently for 21 days becomes a habit.

5. Anything done consistently for 21 days becomes a habit.

6. Anything done consistently for 21 days becomes a habit.

7. Anything done consistently for 21 days becomes a habit.

8. Anything done consistently for 21 days becomes a habit.

9. Anything done consistently for 21 days becomes a habit.

10. Anything done consistently for 21 days becomes a habit.

11. Anything done consistently for 21 days becomes a habit.

12. Anything done consistently for 21 days becomes a habit.

13. Anything done consistently for 21 days becomes a habit.

14. Anything done consistently for 21 days becomes a habit.

15. Anything done consistently for 21 days becomes a habit.

16. Anything done consistently for 21 days becomes a habit.

17. Anything done consistently for 21 days becomes a habit.

18. Anything done consistently for 21 days becomes a habit.

19. Anything done consistently for 21 days becomes a habit.

20. Anything done consistently for 21 days becomes a habit.

21. Anything done consistently for 21 days becomes a habit.

*Journal:*_____

_____

_____

_____

_____

_____

_____

BODY-LIFE NOW!

_____

_____

_____

_____

_____

_____

_____

22. CHALLENGE

Anyone who meets a testing CHALLENGE head-on and manages to stick it out is mighty fortunate. For such persons loyally in love with God, the reward is life and more life. (James 1:12)

⟞⬦⬩⟝

Compete only with yourself

and use your God-given energies to strive for your own, personal best.

There is no easy way to excellence,

no short-cut to success in *any* endeavor, including fitness.

Face and embrace every challenge in your life,

and use your time in the gym, or wherever you train,

to help you prepare for meeting each of them.

Challenges create champions,

and there is a great champion locked up inside you,

ready to be released.

Don't be afraid to take it up a notch.

The next level is unknown territory to you now,

but soon you'll be totally comfortable there, able to do more than you think you can.

And the more that you *do*, the more you *can* do.

Face every challenge head-on.

Don't flinch.

Don't back down.

Feel the fear and *do it anyway.*

Every day is a new and exciting challenge for you to accept and conquer,

and there's a new one waiting for you right now . . .

Go for it!

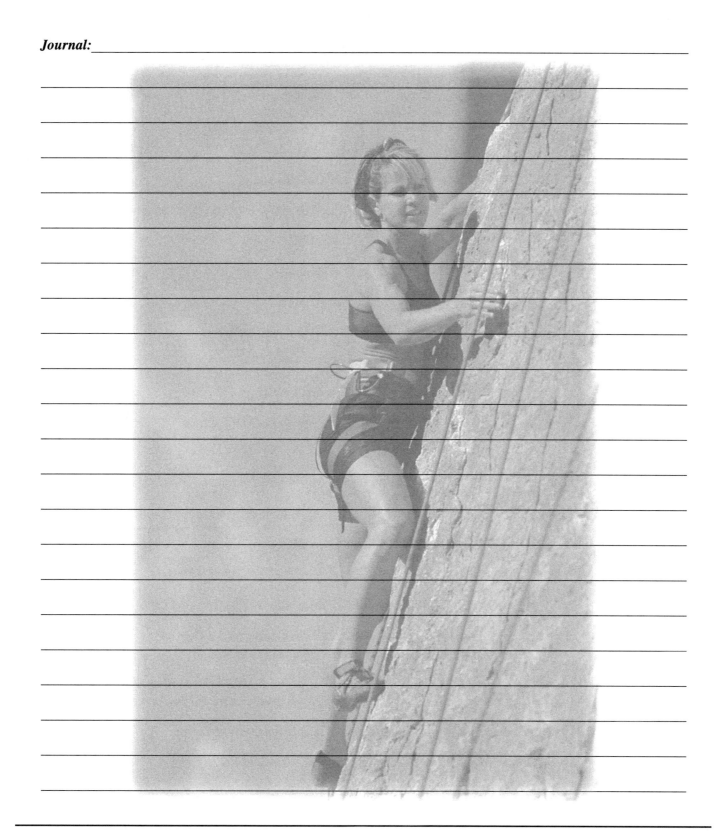

23. VITALITY

My dear lover glows with health – red-blooded, radiant! (Song of Solomon 5:10)

———◆◆———

Your energy is about to kick in.

The very life of God flows through you.

Your strength is *increasing* with age, like that of a tall oak tree that grows stronger through the years.

You glow with a supernatural life force.

God restores the vigor of your youth.

You are lively and quick and animated.

You have a get-up-and-go attitude that keeps you genuinely motivated.

The blessing of your good health is an inspiration to others.

Wellness and wholeness are yours.

You have that extra something that sets you apart from the rest.

You have an edge . . .

a divine spark of life

that keeps you glowing with healthfulness . . . a certain light that shines from within.

You are radiant with the glory of God . . .

strong, muscular, defined,

built up spiritually and physically.

*It stands to reason, doesn't it, that if the alive-and-present God
who raised Jesus from the dead moves into your life,*

*he'll do the same thing in you that he did in Jesus, bringing you alive to himself?
When God lives and breathes in you (and he does, as surely as he did in Jesus),*

you are delivered from that dead life. With his Spirit living in you,

your body will be as alive as Christ's! (Romans 8:11)

*Journal:*_____

BODY-LIFE NOW!

24. COMPETITION

You've all been to the stadium and seen athletes race. Everyone runs; one wins. RUN TO WIN. All good athletes train hard. They do it for a gold medal that tarnishes and fades. You're after one that's gold eternally. (1 Corinthians 9:24,25)

———◆◆———

Run to win, to excel, to triumph!

You were destined to prevail in the arena of life.

For the most part, winning is basically just deciding not to lose,

and then committing to doing what needs to be done to support that decision.

Don't interfere with good people's lives; don't try to get the best of them.

No matter how many times you trip them up, God-loyal people don't stay down long;

Soon they're up on their feet, while the wicked end up flat on their faces.

Don't laugh when your enemy falls; don't crow over his collapse.

God might see, and become very provoked, and take pity on his plight. (Proverbs 24:15-18)

Play hard, but keep it all in perspective.

Give it all you've got, and then know when to let it go.

Find the balance between *winning isn't everything, it's the* only *thing,*

and *it's not whether you win or lose, it's how you play the game.*

In their proper contexts, both statements are true,

and you must find the grace to know how to balance them.

But, without a doubt, winning is good – *very* good.

So train to win.

Visualize yourself as a winner.

Imagine how good it's going to feel to win.

When you fail, get back up as soon as you can and shake it off.

Just do it.

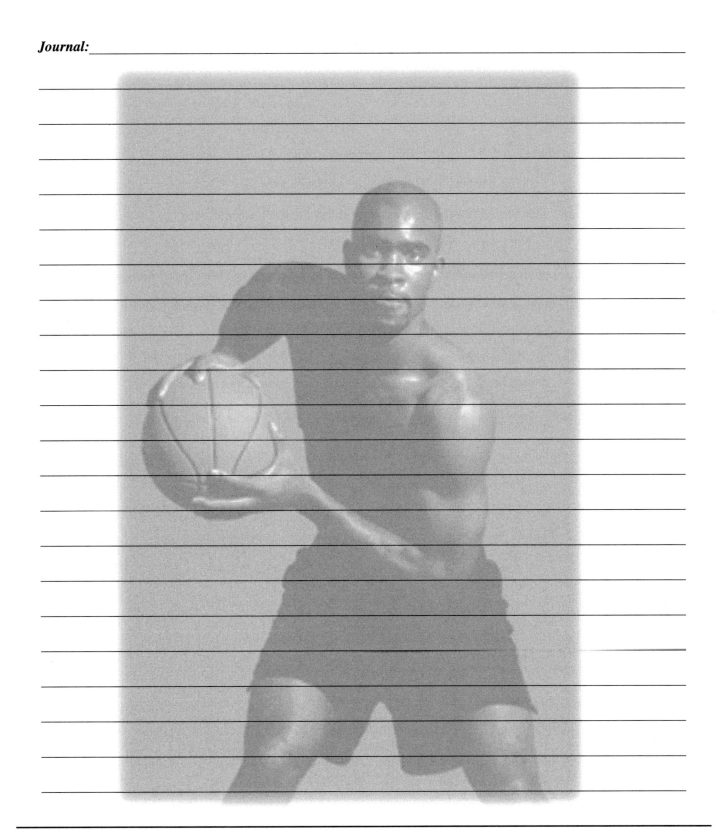

25.   TEAMWORK

So don't sit around on your hands! No more dragging your feet! Clear the path for long-distance runners so no one will trip and fall, so no one will step in a hole and sprain an ankle. Help each other out. And run for it! (Hebrews 12:12,13)

———◆———

A healthy body is the product of teamwork.

What is true for the physical body is true for the Body of Christ.

Meditate on this:

You can easily enough see how this kind of thing works by looking no further than your own body.

Your body has many parts – limbs, organs, cells – but no matter how many parts you can name, you're still one body.

It's exactly the same with Christ . . . A body isn't just a single part blown up into something huge.

It's all the different-but-similar parts arranged and functioning

together. (1 Corinthians 12:12,14)

What is true for the body

is true for every part of your life.

What is true for team sports is symbolic for all living things. No one succeeds alone.

The people on your team, your workout partner, or personal trainer,

all help you get to where you want and need to go.

You need people,

and they need you.

The unity produced by teamwork begins with the individual.

Bringing your spirit, soul and body into oneness is the beginning.

But the *ultimate* teamwork is God and you working *together*.

. . . If God is for us, who can be against us? (Romans 8:31)

Together, you and God form a majority.

*Journal:*_____

BODY-LIFE NOW!

26. ENERGY

. . . Be ENERGETIC in your life of salvation, reverent and sensitive before God. That ENERGY is God's ENERGY, an ENERGY deep within you, God himself willing and working at what will give him the most pleasure. (Philippians 2:12,13)

—•—

You've got the power!

A driving force keeps rising up from the center of your inner self,

and flowing into your muscles and to every fiber of your being.

It is the force of a mighty, raging river,

the same spirit that raised Christ from the dead –

the resurrection life of God Himself.

You are energized to engage in productive movement.

Something *bigger* than you is working *through* you.

Like a magnet to steel, it keeps drawing you back to the gym, or the track, or the field, or the treadmill,

so that you can experience the rush of that burst of energy

that flows from your own vitality.

You anticipate the workout.

You look forward to vigorous exercise.

Your energy overcomes your stress

as you intentionally exhaust your body.

Like a dynamo,

the energy is self-perpetuating and fatiguing at the same time.

The energy is *accessible*.

The energy is *activating*.

The energy is *awesome*.

And as you collapse on the floor, completely spent, you can't wait to do it all over again tomorrow!

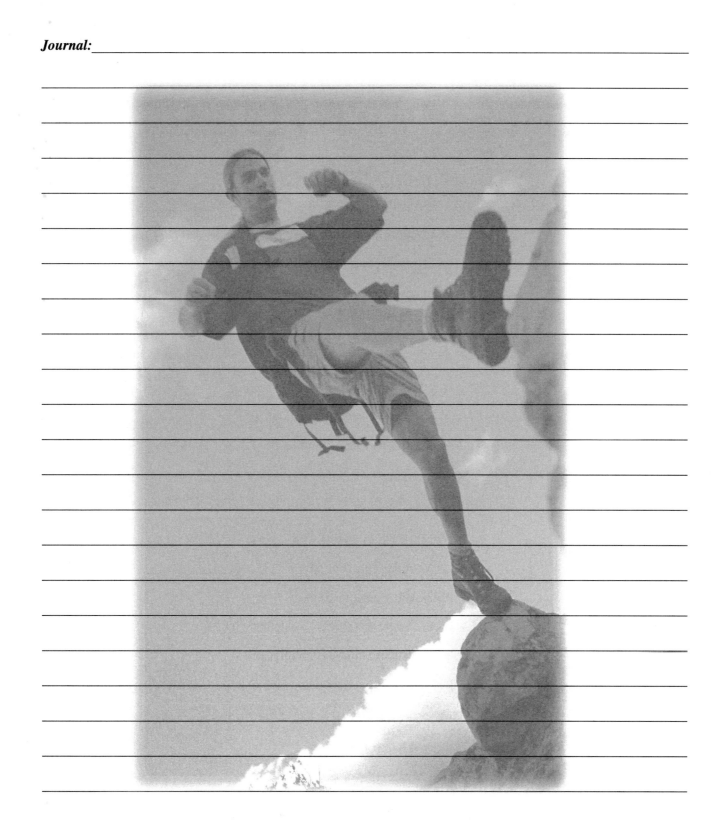

27.   DEVELOPMENT

Then Jesus said, "God's kingdom is like seed thrown on a field by a man who then goes to bed and forgets about it. The seed sprouts and grows – he has no idea how it happens. The earth does it all without his help: first a green stem of grass, then a bud, then the ripened grain. When the grain is fully formed, he reaps – harvest time!" (Mark 4:26-29)

———

Development takes time.

Progress is incremental.

These are facts of nature

and the process of development in the Kingdom of God.

Don't become discouraged if your results are not manifesting as quickly as you would like.

Little by little your body *is* developing into the desired picture of it that you see in your head.

You must be patient.

You must be diligent.

You must be tirelessly committed.

Reward yourself for little victories,

but don't settle for less than what you really want to achieve.

Keep going, no matter what.

Work through your pain.

Maintain a positive attitude.

Avoid negative people who try to discourage you

and pay no attention to their opinions.

Don't give anybody the power over you to affect you in any counterproductive way.

Notice when you see a new "cut" here,

or a new one there.

You *are* developing.

Don't let anyone, including yourself, tell you otherwise.

*Journal:*_____

_____

_____

_____

_____

_____

_____

BODY-LIFE NOW!

_____

_____

_____

_____

_____

_____

_____

_____

_____

28. EMPOWERMENT

. . . God doesn't come and go. God lasts. He's Creator of all you can see or imagine. He doesn't get tired out, doesn't pause to catch his breath. And he knows everything inside and out. He energizes those who get tired, gives fresh strength to dropouts. For even young people tire and drop out, young folk in their prime stumble and fall. But those who wait on God get fresh strength. (Isaiah 40:28-31)

——•◆•——

God has empowered you to take charge of your life and do something positive with it.

You have strength.

You have resources.

You have inspiration.

You have the ability to use your words creatively.

You have the power to determine your progress.

You have the power to believe.

Believe in the power of God in your life.

Believe in yourself.

Believe in your future.

Believe that what you are doing for your physical body is not just a *good* thing –

it is a *necessary* thing.

. . . David strengthened himself with trust in his God. (1 Samuel 30:6)

David was able to do mighty exploits because he knew how to encourage himself in the Lord.

You can encourage yourself, too.

You can strengthen yourself by your own attitude and words.

Speak to your mind.

Speak to your body.

Speak to your circumstances.

Take dominion over your day,

and power it up!

29. FOCUS

Friends, don't get me wrong: By no means do I count myself an expert in all of this, but I've got my eye on the goal, where God is beckoning us onward – to Jesus. I'm off and running, and I'm not turning back. So let's keep FOCUSED on that goal, those of us who want everything God has for us. If any of you have something else in mind, something less than total commitment, God will clear your blurred vision – you'll see it yet! Now that we're on the right track, let's stay on it. (Philippians 3:13-16)

You have a plan, a goal, a strategy.

There is a proven system to fitness, and the information is available to you.

And even though you may be surrounded by unfocused, undisciplined people

who don't have any clear direction for *their* lives

and don't understand what makes *you* tick,

you have to move past them and get busy with your own progress.

You must set the tone for the course of your life.

You must strive to be a "thermostat" rather than a "thermometer." You have the ability to do it.

You can train your mind to train your body.

You know what you want, and you know what you have to do to get it.

Your unbroken focus keeps you from ever becoming discouraged with your results –

you don't have time for discouragement!

A focused mind is a *positive* mind.

A positive mind is a *productive* mind.

A productive mind produces a *fit* body.

A fit body is an integral part of a *successful* life.

Your thoughts are organized

and are translating into an effective workout.

Get the most out of it today . . .

and stay focused.

BODY-LIFE NOW!

30.   GROWTH

. . . My ears are filled with the sounds of promise: "Good people will prosper like palm trees, GROW tall like Lebanon cedars; transplanted to God's courtyard, They'll GROW tall in the presence of God, lithe and green, virile still in old age." (Psalm 92:11-14)

———————

You're growing in strength –

– growing in success

– growing in prosperity.

Where there is life, there is growth.

You are going from glory to glory.

Your muscles are growing.

Your vision is growing.

Your capacity for greatness is growing.

Growth means that you are moving forward.

You know that you can't go back – there is nothing there for you.

You're making progress.

You're advancing every day.

Whether they say it or not, those around you can see it.

You are growing out of a small place,

so that you can move into a larger place.

Growth brings change,

and change is good.

Don't resist it – go with the flow and *grow* with the flow!

You are flourishing.

You are being promoted.

Enjoy the process.

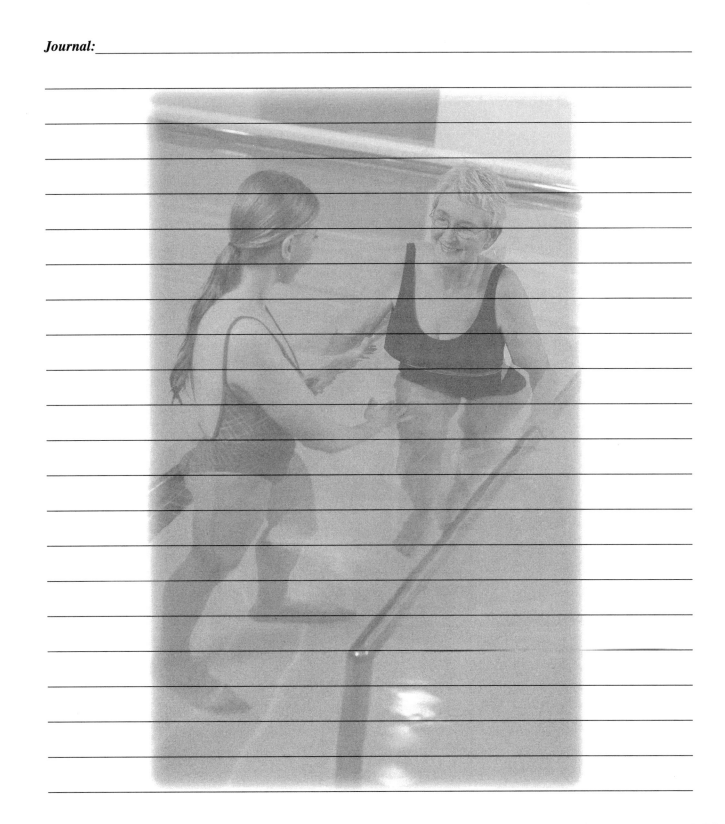

31. CONDITION

I don't know about you, but I'm running hard for the finish line. I'm giving it everything I've got. No sloppy living for me! I'm staying alert and in top CONDITION . . . . (1 Corinthians 9:26,27)

—•◦•—

Getting in shape and staying in shape

requires a deep desire –

– a genuine commitment to personal excellence

– the will to rise to the occasion

– to fearlessly test your limits

by pushing yourself . . .

demanding the *best* from yourself . . .

raising the bar so high that you have to stretch farther than you ever dreamed that you would or could

just to touch the goal.

Conditioning your body enables you, in many ways, to find and free your true self –

to discover that there is much more in you than you have realized up to this point.

It's about unlocking potential.

It's about the power of persistence.

But, conditioning the *mind* is equally important:

Summing it all up, friends, I'd say you'll do best by filling your minds and

meditating on things true, noble, reputable, authentic, compelling, gracious –

the best, not the worst;

the beautiful, not the ugly;

things to praise, not things to curse. (Philippians 3:8)

You can be at the top of your game –

all it takes is conditioning.

---

*Journal:*_____

BODY-LIFE NOW!

32. INCREASE

Clear lots of ground for your tents! Make your tents large. Spread out! Think big! (Isaiah 54:2)

Don't just settle for increasing your muscle mass;

your main goal should be to increase your *vision*.

Your strength is increasing.

Your stamina is increasing.

Every day it gets better.

Every day you move closer to becoming the person that you've always wanted to be.

It's time to think outside the box.

It's time to take on more.

They say, *If you want something done, ask a busy person,*

and *you* have what it takes.

Don't be afraid of success.

Don't be embarrassed to be looked at and admired.

Let your light shine and don't try to hide it.

You can be someone else's inspiration.

Prepare for more.

In your workouts, take it to the next level.

Do a little more.

You are in transition – a season of increase.

You're through the looking glass now.

Get ready for what's coming.

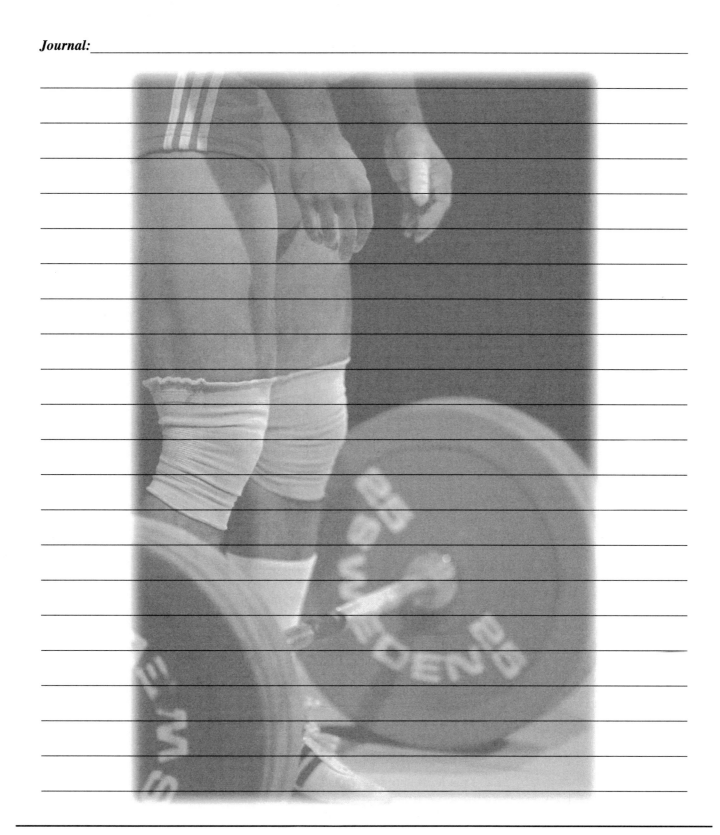

33. INSPIRATION

In this way we are like the various parts of a human body. Each part gets its meaning from the body as a whole, not the other way around. The body we're talking about is Christ's body of chosen people. Each of us finds our meaning and function as a part of his body. But as a chopped-off finger or cut-off toe we wouldn't amount to much, would we? So since we find ourselves fashioned into all these excellently formed and marvelously functioning parts in Christ's body, let's just go ahead and be what we were made to be, without enviously or pridefully comparing ourselves with each other, or trying to be something we aren't. (Romans 12:4-6)

—◆—

Is it worth it? Yes.

Is it in you? Certainly.

Do you have what it takes? Most definitely.

Can you make it? Without a doubt.

Are your goals attainable? For sure.

The functioning of the Body of Christ is your *inspiration*.

The Body of Christ is a champion, and you are a part of that Body.

You can do all things through Christ who strengthens you.

Be encouraged.

Be inspired.

Be blessed.

Can you keep going? So far, so good.

Is it making a difference? You know that it is.

Are you worth the effort? You'd better believe it.

What if you can't maintain the discipline? Don't even go there.

What if you want to quit? That's not an option.

What if you don't feel like it? What's your point?

What if you just don't feel good? Do it anyway.

Can I put it off until tomorrow? Absolutely not.

Go do what you've got to do.

*Journal:*_____

BODY-LIFE NOW!

34. PUSH!

You've made me strong as a charging bison . . . . (Psalm 92:10)

—◆—

Stop complaining and whining and just do it!

There's no need to make excuses;

you know what you need to do, so stop putting it off!

Don't burn out; keep yourselves fueled and aflame . . .

Don't quit in hard times . . . . (Romans 12:11,12)

Come on . . . you know it's time to get busy!

Tell your body what it's going to do.

Don't ask its permission.

Don't consult your feelings.

Stop talking about how tired you are,

or how sore you are,

or how bad the weather is.

None of that matters!

You be the *boss . . . be* somebody!

Push yourself.

Pump up your attitude so that you can pump up your body.

. . . Let the weak say, "I am strong!" (Joel 3:10)

Now is the time.

This is the place.

You've got the power to take it to the limit.

Now, ***PUSH!***

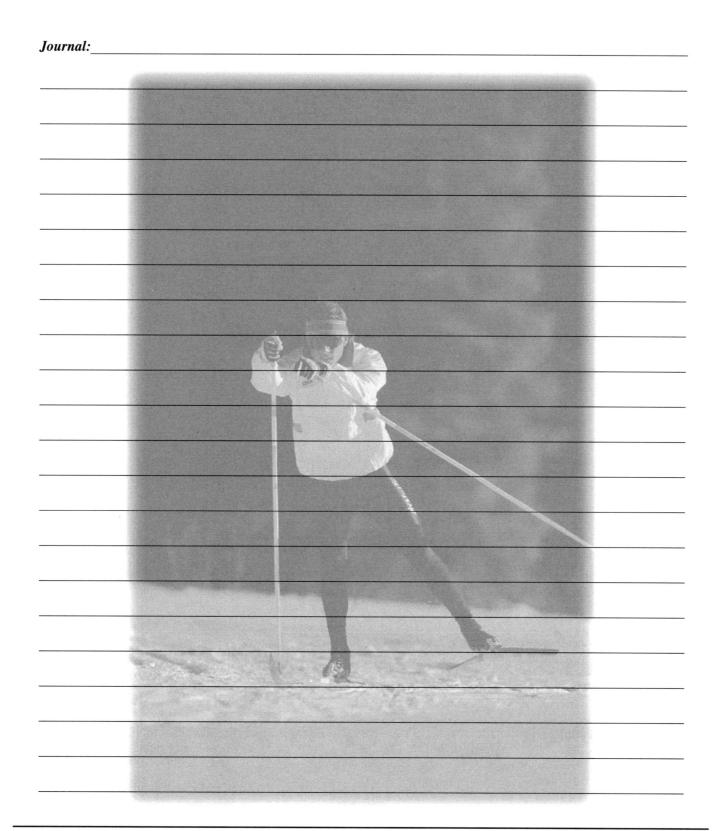

35. CARDIO

Keep vigilant watch over your HEART; that's where life starts. (Proverbs 4:23)

—◆◆—

Developing a heart-healthy attitude is a very important part of creating a winning lifestyle.

In the big picture, when you take care of yourself,

you are really doing a great favor for those who love and need you –

you are serving *them* by preserving your life.

Use whatever stress-reduction techniques work for you.

Change your diet when and if necessary.

Build up your heart with exercise –

to burn calories . . .

to burn fat . . .

to strengthen the muscle.

But the heart that you should be *most* concerned with

is your spirit – your *spiritual* heart.

For out of the abundance of the **heart** *the mouth speaks. A good man out of the good treasure of his* **heart** *brings forth good things, and an evil man out of the evil treasure brings forth evil things. (Matthew 12:34,35)*

So get on that treadmill

or bicycle,

and have yourself a really good cardio workout today.

But don't forget to take care of your *eternal* heart by submitting it to the Word of God.

Wait on the Lord, and He will strengthen your heart.

*Journal:*_____

_____

_____

_____

_____

_____

_____

BODY-LIFE NOW!

_____

_____

_____

_____

_____

_____

36.   MAINTENANCE

A sound mind makes for a robust body, but runaway emotions corrode the bones. (Proverbs 14:30)

——◆——

It's not enough just to *get* there.

The most important thing is learning how to *stay* there.

Discipline is not just something that you pay attention to for a short season of your life;

you're in this for the long-haul.

You're not just trying to lose some weight

or build some muscle.

You are developing a *lifestyle* that you must maintain for the rest of your life.

Your days of dieting are over.

Now you are learning how to *enjoy* eating right, indefinitely.

The hit-or-miss season has ended.

No more dropping out.

No more giving up on yourself.

Now you know how to pace yourself.

You are able to set realistic goals and go after them.

You know how to be accountable to someone – and to yourself.

Most importantly, you are learning the importance of maintaining a good attitude.

And you *must* be diligent to work at the maintenance, because . . .

It's on, now!

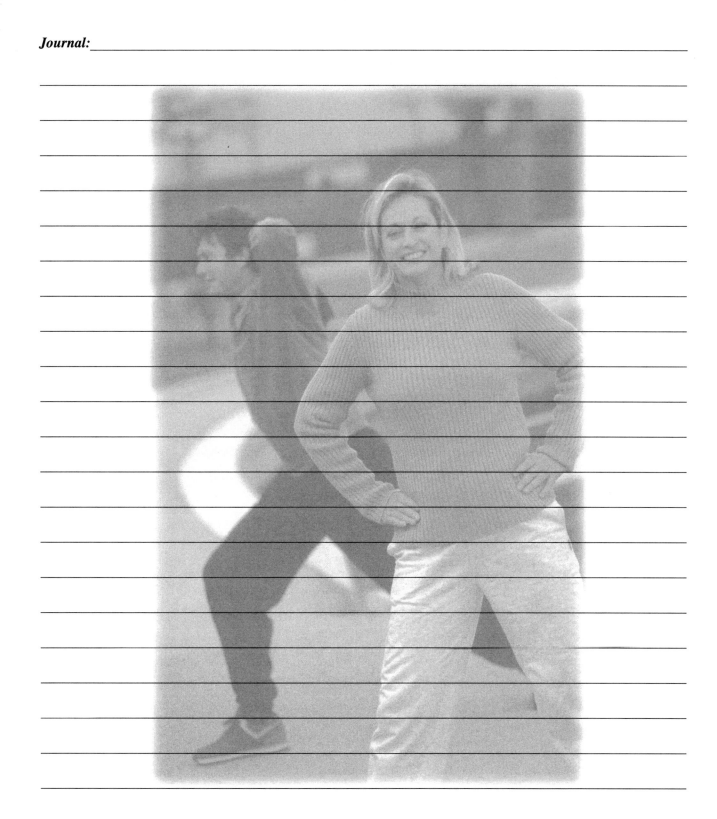

37.   NUTRITION

Only take care, son of man, that you don't rebel like these rebels. Open your mouth and eat what I give you.
(Ezekiel 2:8)

———◆•◆———

You are what you eat. You've heard it said many times, because it's true.

God put such a vast variety of foods for man to eat in His amazing creation,

that we never have to become bored with eating what's good for us.

. . . they'll tell you not to eat this or that food – perfectly good food God created

to be eaten heartily and with thanksgiving by Christians! Everything God created

is good, and to be received with thanks. Nothing is to be sneered at and thrown out.

God's Word and our prayers make every item in creation holy. (1 Timothy 4:3-5)

All the vitamins, minerals, nutrients and proteins that you need are available to you in a healthy diet.

Make good *choices* in your eating today. Don't eat too much or too little.

. . . Give me enough food to live on, neither too much or too little. (Proverbs 30:8)

In this day of celebrated artificiality, it will require a real effort on your part to find natural, whole foods to eat.

But he who seeks will find.

. . . Oh yes, God brings grain from the land,

wine to make people happy,

their faces glowing with health,

a people well-fed and hearty. (Psalm 104:14,15)

To improve the way that you eat, you have to change the way that you think and talk about food.

Be disciplined, without becoming religious and obnoxious about your diet.

But don't let others influence you negatively by causing you to compromise, either.

Nourish yourself by feeding your *whole* self – spirit, soul and body.

Bon appétit!

BODY-LIFE NOW!

38. JUMP!

Look! Listen! There's my lover! Do you see him coming? Vaulting the mountains, leaping the hills.
(Song of Solomon 2:8)

———◆———

Whether on the basketball court, in front of a volleyball net,

or competing in field events . . . long jump, high jump, triple jump, pole vault, hurdles,

it is a gloriously symbolic thing to defy the law of gravity by leaping, unencumbered, into the air above.

From the little girls tirelessly skipping rope on the playground,

to the heavyweight champion of the world doing basically the same thing in his training exercises,

the jump is an expression of man's ability to overcome earth-bound obstacles and soar into the heavens.

But for you, sunrise! The sun of righteousness will dawn on those

who honor my name, healing radiating from its wings.

You will be bursting with energy,

like colts frisky and frolicking. (Malachi 4:2)

Jesus said to jump for joy when you are lied about and persecuted.

His words were more than just the suggestion of a paradigm-shift,

they were the road map to ultimate victory over circumstances.

You are an overcomer!

jUmP fOr JoY!

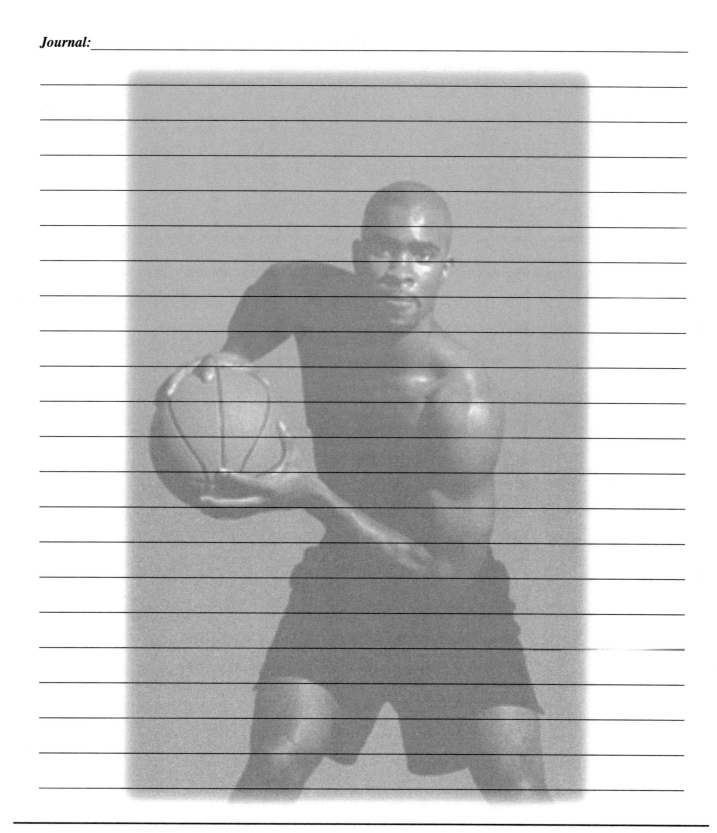

39. STRETCHING

I'm letting you know what I need, calling out for help and LIFTING MY ARMS toward your inner sanctum.
(Psalm 28:2)

—◆◆—

Jesus said to the man with the crippled hand, *"Stretch forth your hand,"*

and when he obeyed, he was healed.

The man was stretching *figuratively* as well as *literally*, because, in doing so, he was reaching for his future.

Stretching is good for muscle tone, increased circulation, prevention of injury, and to promote peaceful relaxation.

But when you stretch before you workout or run, or during a yoga class,

you are affecting the spiritual as well as the physical.

Stretching is *reaching* for something that you can't see in the material world.

It's a way to symbolically enlarge your borders.

. . . my arms wave like banners of praise to you. (Psalm 63:4)

. . . Lord, I have called daily upon You;

I have STRETCHED out my hands to you. (Psalm 88:9)

S-t-r-e-t-c-h toward your better self.

S-t-r-e-t-c-h toward your future.

S – t – r – e – t – c – h out, and possess all of your promised land.

BODY-LIFE NOW!

40. LIFE

Good friend, don't forget all I've taught you; take to heart my commands. They'll help you live a long, long time, a long LIFE lived full and well. (Proverbs 3:1,2)

—◆——◆—

Never take for granted the ability to move and feel and breathe – to be aware – to have a voice . . .

Dear friend, guard Clear Thinking and Common Sense with your life,

don't for a minute lose sight of them. They'll keep your soul alive and well,

they'll keep you FIT and ATTRACTIVE. (Proverbs 3:21,22)

Rejoice that you are still here – that you have not just *survived,* but that you have *thrived!*

Rejoice that you've been given another chance to live your life today.

Dear friend, listen well to my words; tune your ears to my voice.

Keep my message in plain view at all times. Concentrate! Learn it by heart!

Those who discover these words LIVE, really LIVE;

Body and soul, they're bursting with health. (Proverbs 4:20-22)

Take a deep breath. Isn't it wonderful that you can still do that?
Stretch your arms and legs, and realize how *blessed* you are

to have muscles and tendons and joints . . . to have motor skills . . . to have strength.

Live wisely and wisdom will permeate your LIFE;

mock life and life will mock you. (Proverbs 9:12)

Every opportunity that you have to walk or run or stretch or lift is a *blessing* . . . a priceless *gift.*

So stop complaining about the things that you don't like about your body,

and just be thankful today that it is still *alive* after some of the things you've put it through.

Be grateful for what you have to work with and that it still has potential.

Whoever goes hunting for what is right and kind

finds LIFE itself – glorious LIFE! (Proverbs 21:21)

Let all of your physical activity today become a celebration of the miracle of life . . . LIVE every second of this day.

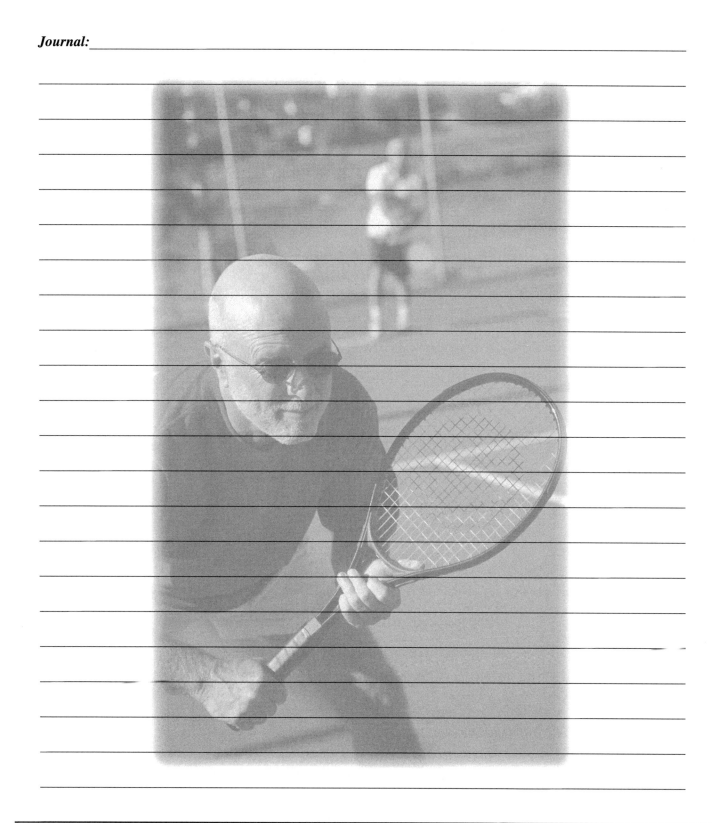

41. AEROBICS

God's Message, the God who created the cosmos, stretched out the skies, laid out the earth and all that grows from it, Who BREATHES life into earth's people, makes them alive with his own life. (Isaiah 42:5)

The point of aerobic exercise is to condition the cardiopulmonary system, by means of vigorous exercise,

in order to increase the efficiency of oxygen intake.

Whatever your preference – an aerobics class, or running, or doing calisthenics –

it's all about the *oxygen* – it's about whole-body *breathing*.

Even the word *exercise* comes from the same root as does *oxygen* . . .

literally, to *exercise* means to "oxygenate" the body.

God created Adam by breathing into him the *breath of life,* so breath is essentially the purest form of creativity.

The word "spirit" is from the Latin *spiritus* (which is literally "breath"),

or *spirare (*"to breathe").

In English, to *inspire* actually means "to breathe into."

Take a deep breath right now.

You just did something good for your brain, for your blood, for your whole body.

Maximize your workout until it affects your breathing . . .

until you are *oxygenated* . . .

until you are *inspired,* even if at the end of it you feel like you are about to *ex*-pire!

Breathe *in* every faith-filled, positive thing . . .

Breathe *out* everything that is negative or cursed.

You are alive and *breathing*!

What could be better than that?

Now go do something aerobic

and let everything that has *breath* praise the Lord!

---

*Journal:*_____

BODY-LIFE NOW!

42. POSSIBILITIES

God can do anything, you know – far more than you could ever imagine or guess or request in your wildest dreams! He does it not by pushing us around but by working within us, his Spirit deeply and gently within us. (Ephesians 3:20)

—◆—

Never say "never."

All things are possible to those who believe.

If you can walk, you can run.

If you can run a 5K race, you can run a 10K race.

If you can run a 10K race, you can run a half-marathon.

If you can run a half-marathon, you can run a marathon.

You can be stronger. Your muscles can be harder. Your body can be leaner.

You can be more flexible. You can be in better shape, internally and externally.

If you can excel *physically*, you can excel *emotionally* and *spiritually*.

Building your body is one way to prove to yourself that you can do just about anything that you really set your mind to.

I have strength for all things in Christ who empowers me

[I am ready for anything and equal to anything through Him Who infuses inner strength into me;

I am self-sufficient in Christ's sufficiency]. (Philippians 4:13 – AMP)

Believe in God.

Believe that He is on your side.

Believe that your dreams can come true.

Believe that all the power you need is already *inside* you.

Believe that your best days are ahead of you.

Believe that you can become the person that you've always wanted to be.

Believe in the opportunities presented to you today.

Your possibilities are unlimited.

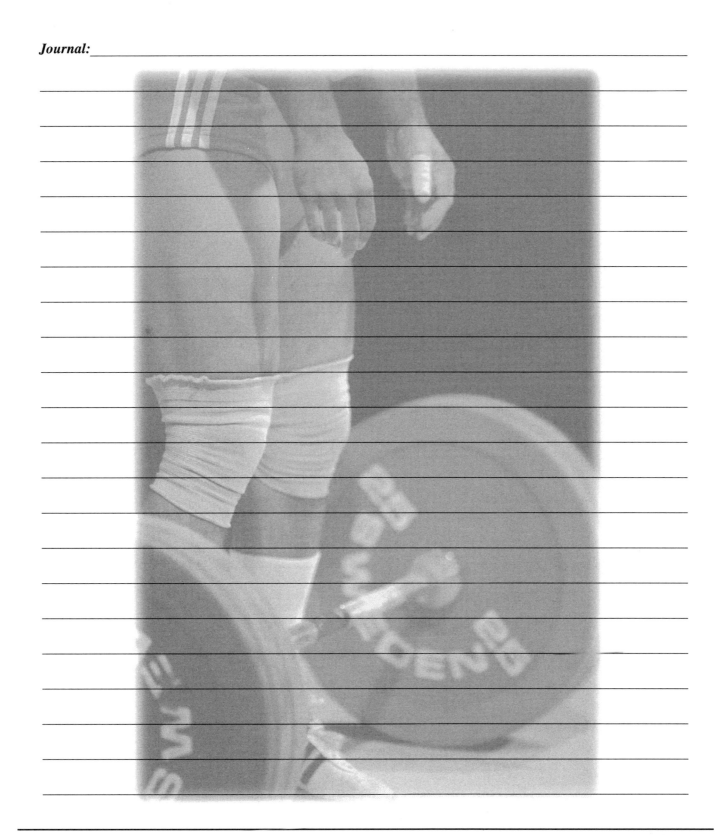

43. ACTION

. . . ACT on what you hear! Those who hear and don't ACT are like those who glance in the mirror, walk away, and two minutes later have no idea who they are, what they look like. (James 1:22-24)

—◆—

Of course a positive mental attitude is important,

but visualization, or wishing, or hoping for a better body, isn't going to increase your muscle mass.

*You **have** to do the work.*

Hiring a personal trainer will never benefit you, unless you commit to doing what he or she tells you to do,

consistently.

Just *talking* about getting in shape is not going to burn one ounce of fat off of you;

you have to spend less time talking, and more time sweating, if you want to move that belt buckle up a notch.

Joining a health club or fitness center will not produce any results for you

unless you actually *use* the facility on a regular basis.

And you can purchase every piece of home gym equipment that money can buy,

but if you only use it to hang your clothes on, you're never going to see your abs.

In the same way, James says about spiritual matters that *faith without **works** is dead.*

Just talking about loving God is not enough.

You have to *do* something to *activate* and *demonstrate* your faith, if you want to have credibility.

If you constantly complain about what you don't like about your body,

but never do anything to improve it, you are lying to yourself.

Never complain about what you permit.

If you mean business, then get busy.

Be proactive.

Take action.

Do it now.

---

*Journal:*_____

_____

_____

_____

_____

_____

_____

BODY-LIFE NOW!

_____

_____

_____

_____

_____

_____

_____

44. CONFIDENCE

The Fear-of-God builds up confidence, and makes a world safe for your children. (Proverbs 14:26)

———•———

Here are the facts about being confident – about having *self*-confidence:

Spirit-filled, virtuous people can and *should* be confident in every area of life.

Believing in yourself does not in any way conflict with your faith or belief in God.

Loving yourself doesn't prevent you from loving *others* – quite the contrary, in fact.

You can absolutely be self-confident and humble at the same time. Jesus was.

Speaking good things about yourself is not the same thing as arrogant bragging.

Pride is only negative when it becomes rebellious self-exaltation.

So don't let anyone convince you that wanting to look better or feel better is just a sign of being egocentric

or self-absorbed.

And don't be naïve enough to confuse confidence with conceit. They are *not* the same thing, at all.

Jesus exuded *total* confidence in everything that He did and said – He believed in Himself, completely –

and, yet, He was *still* the consummate servant and made the ultimate sacrifice for all of mankind.

. . . in quietness and CONFIDENCE shall be your strength. (Isaiah 30:15)

Just be who you *are*, without any apology.

Therefore do not cast away your CONFIDENCE, which has great reward. (Hebrews 10:35)

Work out today with the justified belief that you are becoming the very best that you can be.

Enjoy being *you*.

45. ATTITUDE

Do your best, prepare for the worst – then trust God to bring victory. (Proverbs 21:31)

You've heard it said before that your *attitude* determines your *altitude*, and it does.

Attitude is everything.

Your happiness is not determined by your circumstances –

your happiness is determined by how you *view* your circumstances.

The quality of your workout today will be decided by your attitude toward it.

The people that you encounter today will respond to you according to your attitude.

You have the power to choose your attitude *every* day

and, therefore, you are empowered to create a wonderful life for yourself.

Attitudes are attractive, and a positive outlook and demeanor will attract positive things to you.

Vigorous physical activity can really aid you in shaking off negative feelings

and help you to feel more optimistic about your life and your future.

So, be positive today.

Decide to have a great outlook on the things in your life, keeping them all in perspective.

Be *pro*active, rather than *re*active, to what happens to you.

Choose to walk in joy.

Enjoy the little things – life's simple pleasures – and don't ever take them for granted.

Be happy – regardless of circumstances.

Your attitude will turn the tide and cause things to start working out for your good.

Let bitterness go.

Don't waste your time in self-pity. It's totally counterproductive.

Now, go have a great workout.

*Journal:*_____

_____

_____

_____

_____

_____

_____

_____

_____

_____

BODY-LIFE NOW!

_____

_____

_____

_____

_____

_____

_____

_____

46. SELF-IMAGE

He's not impressed with horsepower; the size of our muscles means little to him. Those who fear God get God's attention, they can depend on his strength. (Psalm 147:10)

━━◆━━

It's good to feel good about your appearance

and to be encouraged with the progress that you're making in reaching your fitness goals.

But don't allow your entire self-image to be wrapped up in the physical.

You have to keep it all in perspective,

or you'll become imbalanced and too self-involved.

As is true with every part of self-improvement,

the most important thing is always to seek *first* the Kingdom of God and His righteousness.

With that principle firmly established in your life,

you can trust yourself to develop a positive, but realistic, view of yourself.

Don't ever feel bad or guilty for wanting to look your best.

You can have a good body self-image and *still* be a nice person . . . and a Christian!

You don't have to justify taking time to do something good for yourself, either,

as long as it is not at the expense of taking care of those for whom you are responsible.

And, by all means, don't allow yourself to maintain a *negative* self-image.

You are who *God* says that you are. Period.

You can do what *God* says that you can do. Period.

You have what *God* says that you have. End of discussion.

As a person, your greatest aim should be to become a good example to others.

Be known for your *character* more than for your physique.

And always walk in faith,

for without it, it is impossible to please God.

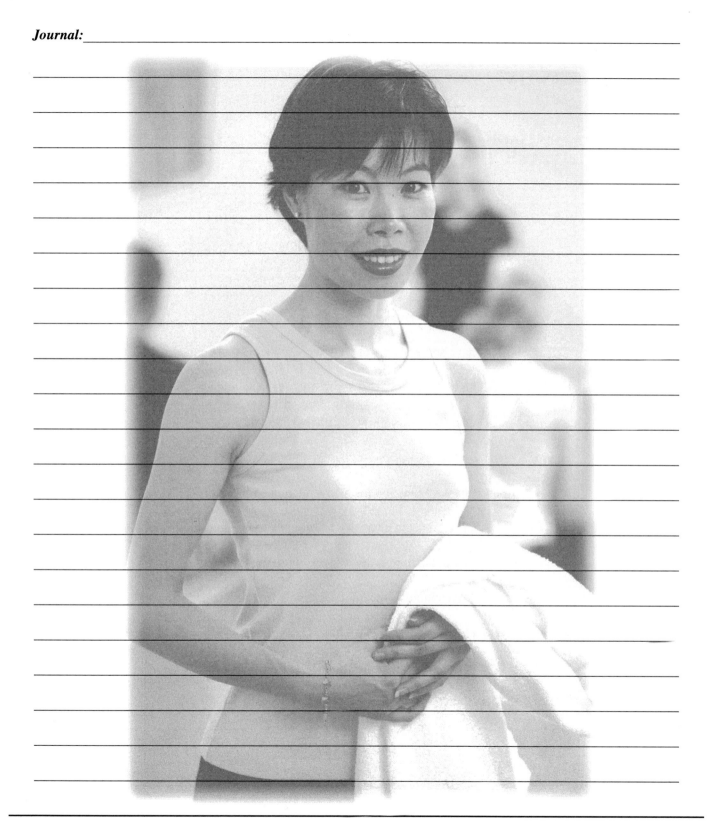

47. LEGS

His LEGS are pillars of marble set on bases of fine gold . . . . (Song of Solomon 5:15)

——◆——

Standing, walking, running, kneeling, bending, kicking, squatting, jumping . . .

your legs make all of that, and more, possible.

Don't dread your leg workout.

It has to be done, so don't waste time by complaining

or by putting it off.

Think of it this way:

your legs have served you well, so you owe them something.

Working out your legs will speed up your metabolism

and increase your overall body strength,

so just do it with a good attitude,

being thankful that you even *have* them to work out.

Your legs are your physical foundation,

and foundation is always very important.

The foundation of your *life* is especially important.

Meanwhile, God's firm foundation is as firm as ever,

these sentences engraved on the stones:

GOD KNOWS WHO BELONGS TO HIM . . . . (2 Timothy 2:19)

*Journal:*_____

_____

_____

_____

_____

_____

_____

BODY-LIFE NOW!

_____

_____

_____

_____

_____

_____

_____

48.   BELIEVE

He touched their eyes and said, "Become what you believe." (Matthew 9:29)

———✦———

Every person eventually becomes what he or she *really* believes that he or she is.

If you don't believe in yourself –

if you don't believe that you can make it –

then you have to change your self-perception,

and you have to get started on it right *now*.

The universe was created by God's faith-filled words,

and He still holds it all together by that same faith.

Faith is the raw material from which every created thing originates,

so, to be God-like, you must be a *believer.*

Believe in your exercise goals.

Believe that they are attainable.

Believe that you are getting stronger every day.

And in your life, believe that God is on your side and that He is working all things together for your good.

Believe that, no matter what may come against you,

after the smoke clears

and the dust settles,

you will still be standing.

Believe in miracles and that they are coming to you right now.

Believe in your potential.

Believe in your gifts.

Believe in today.

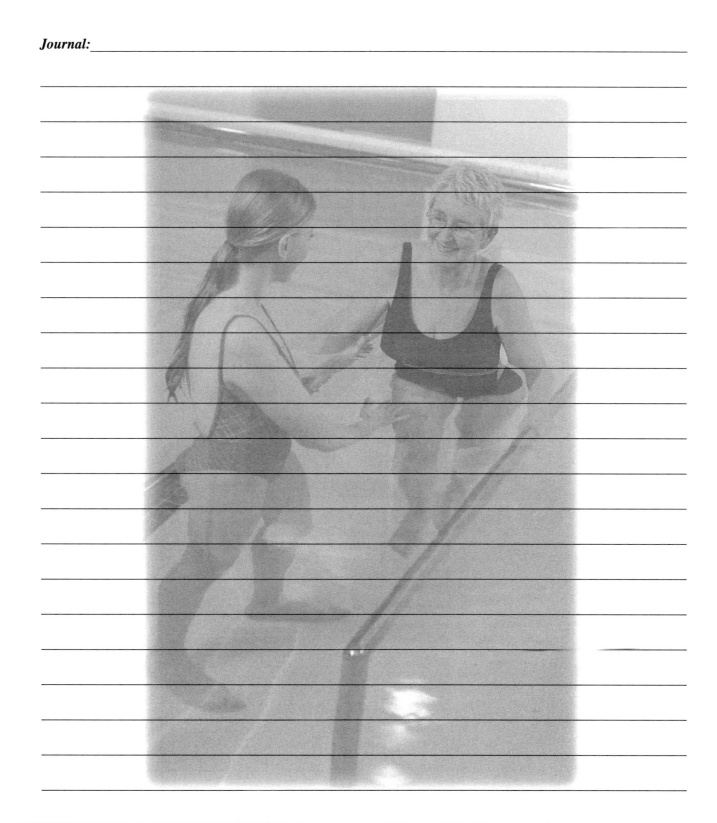

49. ARMS

He shows me how to fight; I can bend a bronze bow! (Psalm 18:34)

———◆———

Your arms are for lifting up in praise toward heaven –

for embracing your loved ones –

for doing the kind of hard work that helps make the world a better place.

Celebrate the strength in your limbs –

your biceps and triceps and forearms.

Pump up your power

and maximize your might with

curls, lifting, push-ups, pull-ups, stretching, pressing . . .

whatever . . .

it's *all* good.

Size, definition, tone, muscularity . . .

they all can be yours

if you stay committed to your workout.

Reach out with those arms

and embrace the bright future that is on its way to you right now.

And remember that God is your strength.

He teaches my hands to make war, so that my ARMS

can bend a bow of bronze. (2 Samuel 22:35)

*Journal:*_____

BODY-LIFE NOW!

50. EXCELLENCE

Trust God from the bottom of your heart; don't try to figure out everything on your own. Listen for God's voice in everything you do, everywhere you go; he's the one who will keep you on track. Don't assume that you know it all. Run to God! Run from evil! Your body will glow with health, your very bones will vibrate with life! (Proverbs 3:5-8)

———

Mediocrity is the enemy of excellence.

Settling for "good enough" will never pave the way to the kind of real excellence that will garner respect.

You are called to greatness,

and the pursuit of it will take you a lifetime.

Success is a journey, not a destination.

Hold yourself to the highest standard possible

and don't allow for any compromise.

Demand *excellence* from yourself.

Expect the *best* from yourself.

Love yourself, but do it with *tough* love.

Don't be too easy on yourself.

Get organized.

Develop a routine.

Keep your word.

Maintain your integrity.

Act like a champion.

Do important things.

Make a real contribution.

Never settle for less than you should.

Live your convictions.

Excel!

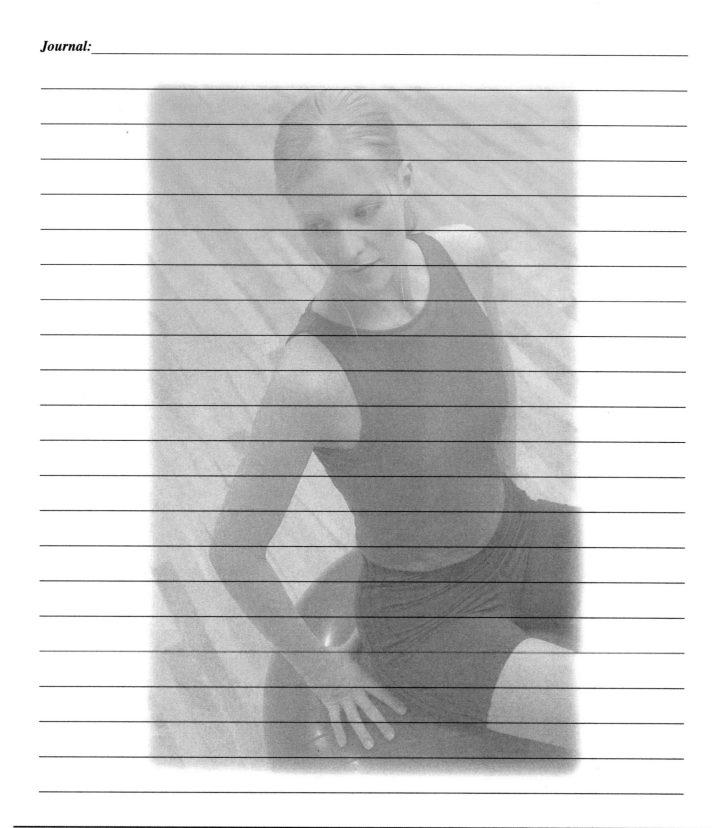

51. SUCCESS

Strength! Courage! . . . Give it everything you have, heart and soul . . . Don't get off track, either left or right, so as to make sure you get to where you're going . . . Then you'll get to where you're going; then you'll SUCCEED. Haven't I commanded you? Strength! Courage! Don't be timid; don't get discouraged. God, your God, is with You every step you take. (Joshua 1:6-9)

———◦•◦———

Success is the ability to *accomplish* – to profit from the power to get things done.

It means being able to start something, and then committing to seeing it through.
It is the use of creativity for a positive and beneficial outcome –

the daily activation of vision . . .

the pursuit of the path of purpose . . .

the navigation of the way of the winner.

Success is a mindset – a way of thinking that produces good results.

It is a self-sustaining lifestyle, because success breeds more success; it produces after its own kind.

Success is a journey, not a destination, and the pursuit of it takes a lifetime.

It is developed through trial and error . . . through a process of learning how to be proactive in every situation.

Success empowers you to move beyond just taking care of yourself,
so that you can bless and improve the world around you.

To be successful, you must value the integrity of your own word – to do what you *say* you will do.

You must make a deep and sincere commitment to maintaining excellence in every area of your life.

Successful people live in the *now*.

They don't waste their precious time with thoughts of regret over the past

or anxiety about the future.

Success is basically a decision – one that must be made daily.

Make the decision to succeed right now, and then walk in all the light that you have at this moment.

Your body will soon begin to show signs of success in your fitness training.

Keep going in the right direction,

and take pride in what you have accomplished.

*Journal:*_____

BODY-LIFE NOW!

52. ABS

Listening to gossip is like eating cheap candy; do you really want junk like that in your BELLY?
(Proverbs 18:8)

⸺⬦⸺

It's no wonder that the words "belly" and "heart" are used interchangeably in the Scriptures.

In their proper contexts, they both have to do with the *center* of a person.

When you work your abdominal muscles –

sit-ups, crunches, whatever –

you are targeting your physical *center*.

You have a *spiritual* center that is referred to in Scripture as *the innermost parts of the belly.*

You have a *soul*-ish or intellectual center, which is the deepest part of your mind –

the source of every deep and important thought.

And you have a *physical* center, which is your abdominal area.

When you work your abs, you are doing more than just trying to flatten your front section

or sculpt a "six-pack."

You are dealing with the *center* of your physique,

and that gives that area of your body great importance and significance.

Don't give up on your quest for well-defined abs.

You will have to do the *work* to burn the fat,

and you'll have to watch what you eat,

but the results will be well worth it.

The more muscle you develop in that area, the more *centered* you will become physically.

But don't forget to keep your heart and mind centered, as well.

Remember, you are a *whole* person.

Now, go do another set of crunches.

*Journal:*_____

53. CONTROL

So don't lose a minute in building on what you've been given, complementing your basic faith with good character, spiritual understanding, alert discipline, passionate patience, reverent wonder, warm friendliness, and generous love, each dimension fitting into and developing the others. (2 Peter 1:5-7)

<hr/>

To get the most out of your weightlifting, you must concentrate on maintaining *control* of the weights.

Proper control helps to promote strength building and definition and also helps you with your coordination.

The *way* that you lift is equally as important as how *much* you lift.

Being physically fit is one very powerful way to take control of your *life*.

Being in control means that you *tell* your body what to do –

that you train it regularly, regardless of how it feels.

Being in control means being disciplined in your diet.

It means eating what you *need*, rather than just eating what you *want*.

Control means that *you* are running your life, instead of your life running you.

People who allow their lives to get out of control, rarely, if ever, accomplish great things.

So, take charge of your life

and, in taking charge of your life, take charge of your workout.

Pay attention to the way that you move when you lift the weights.

Take control over the rhythm and movement of each set.

Use the power in your body to dominate the weight.

You are in control.

You are in charge.

You are calling the shots.

The fruit of the Spirit is . . . self-control . . . . (Galatians 5:22-23)

You have the power to give God the control of your life,

and that decision will be the wisest one that you will ever make.

*Journal:*_____

BODY-LIFE NOW!

54. KNEES

Energize the limp hands, strengthen rubbery KNEES. (Isaiah 35:3)

———

Knees were made for kneeling in prayer and worship,

but they are essential for all physical activity.

Exercise, hydration and good nutrition are beneficial for bones and joints –

Your body will glow with health,

your very BONES will vibrate with life! (Proverbs 3:8) –

and life-giving words produced by a positive mind are good for the bones, as well –

. . . a good report makes the BONES healthy. (Proverbs 15:30)

Take good care of your knees – you're going to need them for a lifetime.

Drink lots of water.

Take your vitamins.

Make sure you get enough calcium in your diet.

Stay positive.

Pleasant words are like a honeycomb, sweetness to the soul and health to the BONES. (Proverbs 16:24)

A joyful attitude conditions your joints and helps to keep you feeling young.

A merry heart does good, like a medicine, but a broken spirit dries the BONES. (Proverbs 17:22)

The name of arthritis must bow to the name of Jesus.

By His stripes you are healed.

Journal: _____

_____

_____

_____

_____

_____

_____

_____

_____

_____

_____

_____

_____

_____

_____

_____

_____

_____

_____

_____

55. REHABILITATION

As for you, I'll come with healing, curing the incurable . . . . (Jeremiah 30:17)

———✦———

Good news! There is hope for the total restoration of your body!

If you have suffered an injury, or have had to undergo surgery,

you *can* be completely rehabilitated through physical therapy –

by taking good care of your body –

by diligently following your doctor's orders –

by proper nutrition –

by practicing temperance (self-control), by being patient –

and by keeping a positive mental attitude.

Most importantly, you can be restored by using your *faith* to help yourself recover.

Believe in and *claim* the promise that you *will* be well again –

. . . your HEALING shall spring forth speedily . . . . (Isaiah 58:8)

Meditate on the Word of God concerning your recovery –

Those who discover these words live, really live;

body and soul, they're bursting with HEALTH. (Proverbs 4:22)

Speak to your body, using the creative force in your tongue to take dominion over your pain and weakness.

Tell your body what it has to do, and expect it to comply.

Death and life are in the power of the tongue . . . . (Proverbs 18:21)

When a broken bone mends, it becomes twice as strong as it was before the break.

That's the way it can be with your whole body . . .

your latter will be greater than your former.

Don't lose your vision for a *complete* restoration.

*Journal:*_____

BODY-LIFE NOW!

56. DOMINION

God created human beings; he created them godlike, reflecting God's nature. He created them male and female. God blessed them: "Prosper! Reproduce! Fill Earth! Take Charge!" (Genesis 1:27,28)

———◆—◆———

Be strong in the Lord, and in the power of His might.

You can do all things through Christ Who strengthens you.

If God is for you, who can be against you?

In all these things you are more than a conqueror.

Greater is He Who is in you, than he who is in the world.

He has made you the head and not the tail,

above only, and not beneath.

You walk by faith, and not by sight.

The wicked flee when no man pursues, but the righteous are as bold as a lion.

You can run through a troop and leap over a wall.

The Lord is the strength of your life.

Let the weak say, "I am strong!"

The joy of the Lord is your strength.

You have the mind of Christ.

You are blessed when you come in, and blessed when you go out.

The Lord compasses you with favor as with a shield.

The angel of the Lord encamps 'round about you.

The Lord gives you the power to get wealth, that He may establish His covenant with you.

This is the day that the Lord has made.

These are the promises of God to *you*.

Now, go *do* something with them. Take dominion!

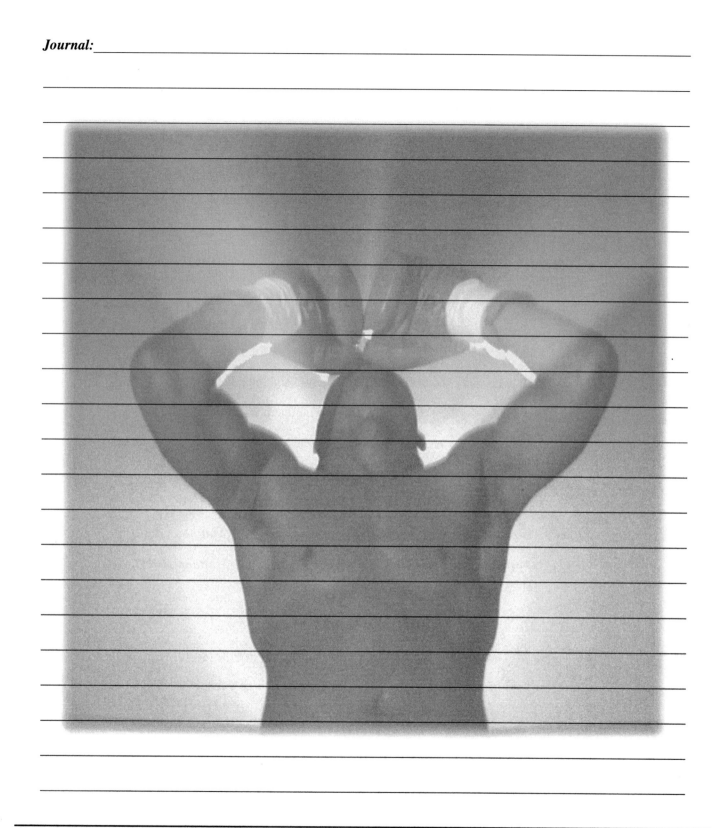

57. PARTNERS

It's better to have a PARTNER than go it alone. Share the work, share the wealth. And if one falls down, the other helps, but if there's no one to help, tough! (Ecclesiastes 4:9,10)

———◆———

A workout partner is a great thing to have.

Having someone to walk, run, or exercise with makes the activity much easier and considerably more enjoyable.

A partner demands accountability of you.

It's easier to get up early and go to the gym when you know that someone is meeting you.

"Hey, buddy, will you spot me?" These are words you say to someone that you can trust.

Covenant is *always* a matter of trust.

Covenant helps you take your commitment to a deeper level –

and everything about the Kingdom of God is about covenant.

A partner speaks words of encouragement to you that help you keep going,

and this is a principle straight from the heart of God:

TWO are better than one . . . . (Ecclesiastes 4:9)

Can TWO walk together, unless they are agreed? (Amos 3:3)

Where TWO or three are gathered together in My name . . . . (Matthew 18:20)

. . . if TWO of you agree on earth concerning anything . . . . (Matthew 18:19)

If you want a partner, *ask* for one,

and then put forth the effort to *connect*.

A man who has friends must himself be friendly . . . . (Proverbs 18:24)

Have you told your workout partner lately how much you appreciate him/her?

*Journal:*_____

_____

_____

_____

_____

_____

_____

_____

BODY-LIFE NOW!

_____

_____

_____

_____

_____

_____

_____

_____

58.   MEDITATION

Summing it all up friends, I'd say you'll do best by filling your minds and MEDITATING on things true . . . .
(Philippians 4:8)

———•+•———

Meditation is good for your spirit, soul, and body.

But his delight is in the law of the Lord, and in His law he MEDITATES day and night.

He shall be like a tree planted by the rivers of water, that brings forth its fruit in its season,

whose leaf also shall not wither; and whatever he does shall prosper. (Psalm 1:2,3)

Meditation is not weird, or cultic, or strange.

Let the words of my mouth

and the MEDITATION of my heart

be acceptable in Your sight O Lord, my strength and my Redeemer. (Psalm 19:14)

Meditation in the Word of God produces prosperity and success:

This book of the law shall not depart from your mouth,

but you shall MEDITATE in it day and night,

that you may observe to do according to all that is written in it.

For then you will make your way prosperous, and then you will have good success. (Joshua 1:8)

Meditation is a devotional exercise of contemplation

that produces positive physical results.

It is reflection.

It is pondering.

It causes the spirit to digest truth in the way that the body digests food.

It is beneficial.

It promotes health.

It is something you should do regularly without reservation.

59. VARIETY

Forget about what's happened; don't keep going over old history. Be alert, be present. I'm about to do something brand-new. It's bursting out! Don't you see it? (Isaiah 43:18,19)

—————⟫•⟪—————

It's good for your body and mind to periodically change your workout routine.

Mixing it up a little shocks your muscles in a positive way and gives you better results.

Change is good.

Do something different.

Dialogue with others about what *they* do.

Expose yourself to new information.

Think outside the box.

Do something you haven't done before.

Change positions when lifting weights to affect a different part of the muscle.

If you walk or run outside, go a different way or direction than normal.

Find new ways to do your cardio workout.

Consider working out at a different time than usual – at least occasionally.

Go buy something new to wear when you work out. It might inspire you to do better.

In the gym, try using a machine you've never used before.

Take a class that you've never taken.

Ask someone what they are doing that is working for them.

Get out of your rut.

Break your cycle.

Transcend your plateau.

Maybe God is about to do something new in your life,

and embracing variety can help you to prepare for it!

*Journal:*_____

BODY-LIFE NOW!

60. SERENITY

God, my shepherd! I don't need a thing. You have bedded me down in lush meadows, you find me quiet pools to drink from. True to your word, you let me catch my breath and send me in the right direction. (Psalm 23:1-3)

Be quiet in your spirit . . . think peaceful thoughts . . . take some deep breaths . . .

calm yourself down . . . let the stress go . . . shake off every negative thing that has attached itself to you . . .

maintain your emotional balance . . . choose your battles wisely . . . remember,
you do not wrestle with flesh and blood.

Remain centered within yourself – you dwell in the secret place of the Most High
and abide under the shadow of the Almighty.

Focus on what is most important right now.

Allow yourself to be refreshed in the Spirit.

Don't let yourself become agitated, anxious, or fretful.

Stop worrying, because worry will not and cannot change things.

Let go of your F.E.A.R. (**F**alse **E**vidence **A**ppearing **R**eal) . . . you have power, love, and a sound mind!

Reckon yourself one with God, and one with yourself.

Be made whole – spirit, soul and body – you are complete in Him.

Allow your sense of self to flow from God's perspective.

The gift of well-being is yours today . . .

open your eyes to all the beauty around you . . . open your soul to all the people who love you . . .

you are experiencing transformation, as you go from glory to glory.

Walk in the light.

Receive with gladness the gift of P.E.A.C.E. (**P**lace **E**very **A**nxiety on **C**hrist, **E**ntirely)

Meditate on all the promises of God.

Enjoy your exercise or walk or workout.

Be at peace in your body, as well as in your spirit.

Let not your heart be troubled . . .

*Journal:*_____

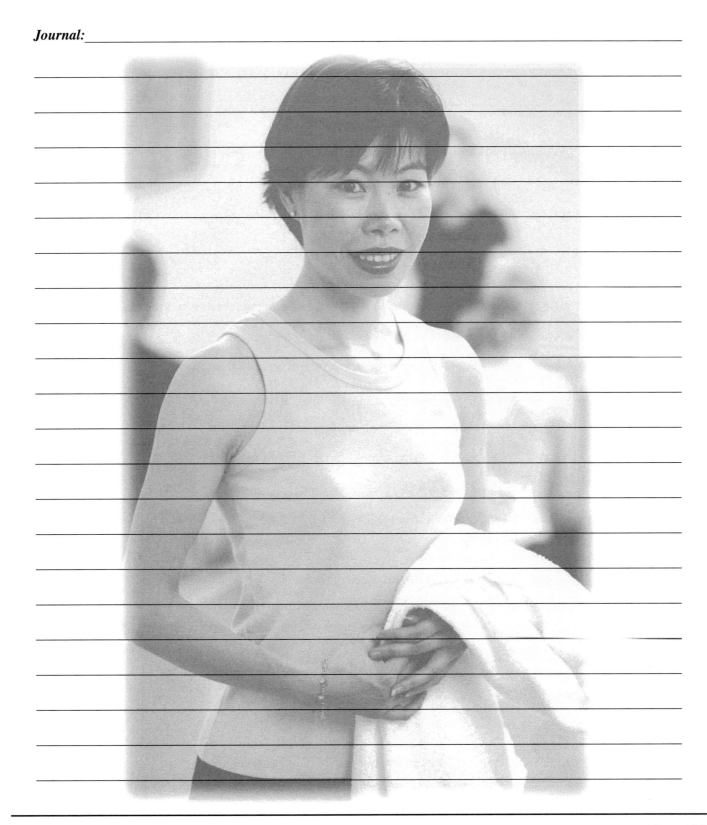

61. FITNESS

A twinkle in the eye means joy in the heart, and good news makes you feel FIT as a fiddle.
(Proverbs 15:30)

———◆———

Your health is a precious gift that should be cherished, protected, and never taken for granted.

Strength training improves the quality of your life, and may even prolong it.

Getting in shape, and staying in shape, is a worthy goal and one that should be pursued for a lifetime

because, ultimately, it is the pursuit of *excellence*.

Fitness is not just about developing your muscles.

The *big picture* involves much more than simply working out on a regular basis.

Fitness is about learning to be disciplined in a way that can positively affect *every* area of your life.

Fitness is training the body as a direct result of successfully training the mind.

Fitness is developing physical endurance so that you can live a much more productive life.

Fitness is about increasing your stamina for your survival in the real world.

Fitness is making a commitment to your future.

Fitness is about daring to be the best that you can be.

It means having the self-esteem that is needed to enjoy a winning lifestyle.

Fitness is for champions.

It increases confidence . . .

elevates self-image . . .

promotes wellness . . .

enables you to rethink yourself . . .

creates a transformation inside and out.

Fitness is power –

power that is worth pursuing.

*Journal:*_____

BODY-LIFE NOW!

62.   DEDICATION

Indolence wants it all and gets nothing; the energetic have something to show for their lives.
(Proverbs 13:4)

———◆◆———

You must be dedicated if you want to attain your goals.

You can't just work out every now and then and expect your body to be anything but *sore*!

Anything worth doing is worth doing *well,*

and nothing can be done well without dedication.

I beseech you therefore, brethren, by the mercies of God,

that you PRESENT YOUR BODIES a living sacrifice, holy, acceptable to God,

which is your reasonable service. (Romans 12:1)

Put your whole heart into your workout.

Make the commitment to be consistent, even when it is not convenient for your schedule.

Be loyal to *yourself,* so that you can keep working to overcome your physical obstacles

to make your body do what you want it to do.

Be single-minded . . .

A double minded man is unstable in all his ways. (James 1:8 - KJV)

More importantly,

dedicate your *life* to something bigger than yourself . . .

to a worthy cause . . .

to God!

An undedicated life is a hollow one.

You have to believe in yourself . . .

in *your* purpose . . . in *your* destiny . . .

in *your* dedication.

Journal:

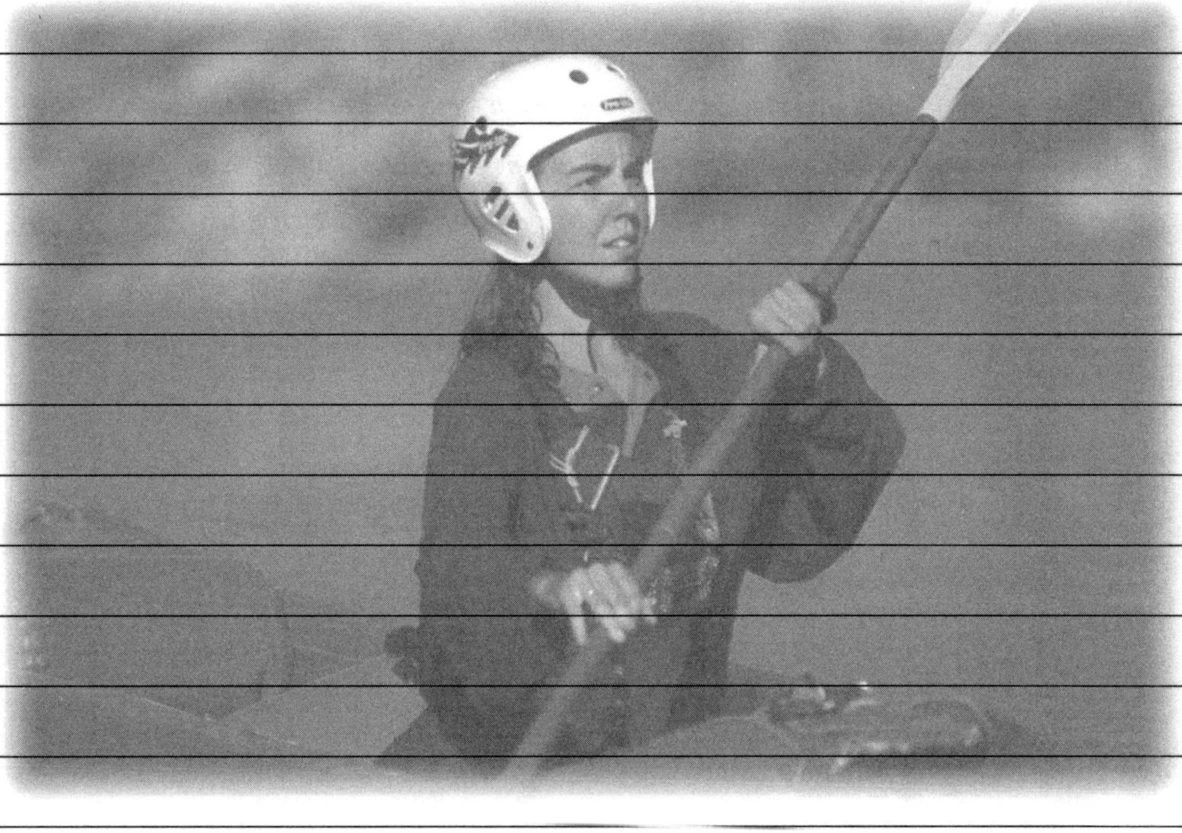

63. WORDS

Gracious speech is like clover honey – good taste to the soul, quick energy for the body.
(Proverbs 16:24)

———•——•———

Words are the building blocks of the universe.

God created His worlds by the words of His mouth –

you create *your* world by the words of *your* mouth.

Your words definitely affect your ability to manage your body:

For we all often stumble and fall and offend in many things. And if anyone

does not offend in speech [never says the wrong things] he is a fully developed

character and a perfect man, ABLE TO CONTROL HIS WHOLE BODY

and to curb his entire nature. (James 3:2 - AMP)

You have what you say, if you believe in your heart that what you say will come to pass.

Don't curse your body by continually talking about what you think is wrong with it.

Speak of your physique as if it already is the way that you would like for it to be.

Your body will eventually begin to conform to your words.

You can't have a good workout if you spend the whole time talking about how *bad* you feel.

If you don't have something good to say, just be quiet and get started.

It's important to talk *up* your workout

and to accentuate the positive about your results.

The more you speak about your excellent health, the healthier you will become.

Start your exercise by saying how *good* you feel (even if you don't) . . .

and how much you are looking forward to it.

You'll be amazed at how great you actually *will* start to feel after a few minutes of getting busy.

Make your words work for you today.

Journal: _____

_____

_____

_____

_____

_____

_____

BODY-LIFE NOW!

_____

_____

_____

_____

_____

_____

64.   MASSAGE

. . . they will lay hands on the sick and make them well. (Mark 16:18)

———◆·▬———

Touch heals.

Jesus, the "Healer of Galilee," had a ministry of *touch*.

He was touchable, and He was *in* touch with hurting people.

He instituted the laying on of hands for the healing of diseases.

He washed His disciples' feet.

A woman washed *His* feet with her hair.

Another woman said, "If I can *touch* His clothes, I shall be made well."

He made mud with His saliva, and put it on a blind man's eyes to heal him.

The Apostle John physically leaned on Him at the Last Supper.

He commanded Thomas to feel the wounds in His hands and side after the resurrection.

His ministry was very tactile and quite physical.

The healing arts that involve touch can be very beneficial for your spirit, soul and body . . .

chiropractic care . . .

reflexology . . .

the various forms of massage. . .

each of these can literally work miracles

for your aching back,

as well as for your stressed-out mind.

Massage can improve muscle tone, and relieve depression at the same time.

So go ahead and treat yourself.

You're worth it.

And keep in touch!

65. TODAY

Give your entire attention to what God is doing right now, and don't get worked up about what may or may not happen tomorrow. God will help you deal with whatever hard things come up when the time comes. (Matthew 6:34)

———•———

Carpe Diem!

Seize the day!   Seize *this* day!

This is *your* day – *your* opportunity – to do something good for your body and for your life.

Don't put off physical activity –

procrastination will never pump up your pecs!

Never let yesterday use up today . . .

let yesterday go . . .

get into the *now*!

There's no time like the present to make a positive difference.

And stop being so distracted by the future . . .

Take no thought for tomorrow . . .

tomorrow will be here soon enough,

with a whole *new* set of circumstances for you to deal with.

What you have is right *now*,

so don't miss this opportunity to improve yourself.

And, by all means, *enjoy* the day!

Make the most of everything that happens to you in these 24 hours.

See your glass half full, and be thankful for all of your blessings.

You have a life to live.

You have *time*.

You have *today*!

Journal: _____

_____

_____

_____

_____

_____

_____

_____

BODY-LIFE NOW!

_____

_____

_____

_____

_____

_____

_____

_____

66.   ENDURANCE

Consider it a sheer gift, friends, when tests and challenges come at you from all sides. You know that under pressure, your faith-life is forced into the open and shows its true colors. So don't try to get out of anything prematurely. Let it do its work so you become mature and well-developed, not deficient in any way.
(James 1:2-4)

Fame can come in a moment, but greatness comes with *longevity*.

Every day that you work out, or run, or exercise, you are challenging your endurance one more time.

The pursuit of physical fitness continually puts your will to the test.

Your strength is proven again and again.

Endurance requires proper maintenance of your *body* –

. . . consistency in your routine,

. . . power-charging your body with optimum nutrition,

. . . getting enough quality rest and hydration.

Endurance is important in your *life*, as well.

All those sayings about enduring through hard times may sound cliché,

but they are absolutely true:

When the going gets tough, the tough get going.

Tough times don't last, but tough people do.

What doesn't break you, will make you.

The force of patience applied to your workout – or to your *life* –

will gradually cause you to evolve into a tower of strength.

Make the choice to endure, no matter how challenging your circumstances may be.

Through faith and patience [we] inherit the promises. (Hebrews 6:12)

Through the process of time, you are becoming stronger than you ever thought you could be.

Don't *ever* give up!

Go the distance!

67.   DISCOURAGEMENT

So let's not allow ourselves to get fatigued doing good. At the right time we will harvest a good crop if we don't give up, or quit. (Galatians 6:9)

Be encouraged!

You *are* making progress, whether you can see it or not.

Don't even *think* about quitting. You've put too much time into reaching your goals
to ever consider ending your pursuit.

You are on a quest, and there's no turning back.

Don't be discouraged with that part of your body that *still* doesn't look or feel like you want it to.

It just takes time, and that's all there is to it.

Walking by faith is refusing to be moved by what you see.

The image in your mirror,

or the number that you see on the scales when you weigh yourself,

are just temporary things.

They are not the last word concerning your physical condition.

You must keep your eye on the prize and refuse to waver from your path.

Overcome any discouragement that you may have by being proactive . . .

by working harder . . .

by giving yourself an attitude adjustment.

Your progress may be incremental,

but it is not imagined.

You really *have* come a long way,

so stop feeling sorry for yourself,

shake it off,

and *do* what you've got to do!

---

*Journal:*_____

BODY-LIFE NOW!

---

68. HEALTH CLUB

So let's **do** *it – full of belief, confident that we're presentable inside and out. Let's keep a firm grip on the promises that keep us going. He always keeps his word. Let's see how inventive we can be in encouraging love and helping out, not avoiding worshipping together as some do but spurring each other on . . . .*
(Hebrews 10:22-25)

You're very fortunate if you have a good fitness center or gym available for your use.

A health club or spa can be a place that provides great inspiration for you in the pursuit of your fitness goals.

The camaraderie that you can enjoy with other people who are on the same page with you

creates a positive and motivational environment that makes it easier to keep up the pace.

You are surrounded by people who are trying to improve themselves,

and, intentionally or unintentionally, they provide valuable encouragement for your own program.

There is also an accountability issue to be considered.

When you make the commitment to pay for a membership at a fitness center,

you are much more likely to take your working out seriously.

You *could* work out on your own at home, but the probability is that you will not –

at least not consistently.

People need to be involved in a local church for much the same reason.

You certainly *can* and *should* pray and read the Bible privately, and on your own,

but the likelihood is that you will not – at least not consistently.

The genuine commitment to attending regular church services

is insurance that you will pay more attention to spiritual things.

So utilize your local gym if you want to maximize your potential. Make the investment in yourself.

Don't let your membership lapse. Get into a regular routine.

Your health club is a great place to develop relationships with like-minded people.

Do it for yourself.

And be an inspiration to somebody else.

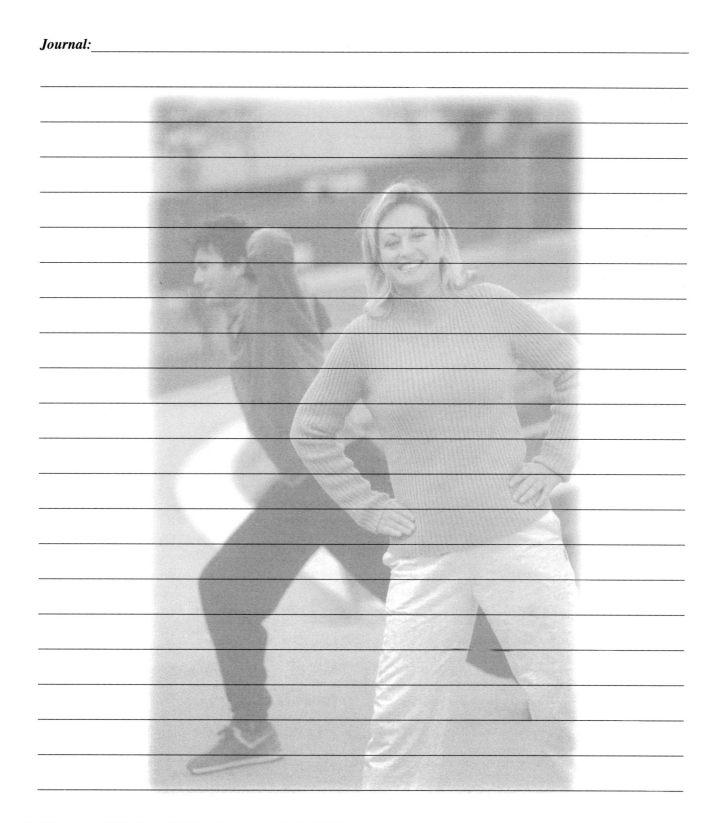

69. ATHLETICS

And also if anyone competes in ATHLETICS, he is not crowned unless he competes according to the rules.
(2 Timothy 2:5)

———◆———

Playing sports and enjoying athletic competition is not just a fun way to get a good workout.

Many valuable life-lessons can be learned from engaging in them: fairness, team mentality, commitment, integrity, etc.

Play a game of baseball or softball. It's not just the great American national pastime,

it's an exercise in the values that cause greatness in life. Healthy competition is good for your psyche.

And there's nothing better for you than enjoying a good swim:

And He will spread out His hands in their midst

as a SWIMMER reaches out to SWIM . . . . (Isaiah 25:11)

or showing your skills on a basketball court:

Blessed shall be your BASKET . . . . (Deuteronomy 28:5)

Golf may be your game – or tennis, or racquetball –

it's *all* good.

Any form of boxing – from kickboxing to simply pounding on a punching bag –

is a great stress reliever,

as are any of the various martial arts.

Therefore I do not run uncertainly [without definite aim]. I do not

BOX as one beating the air and striking without an adversary. But

[like a BOXER] I buffet my body [handle it roughly, discipline it

by hardships] and subdue it . . . . (1 Corinthians 9:26,27 - AMP)

Go throw around the football or get into a vigorous game of table tennis.

Athletics provide so many great ways to get exercise that you never have to run out of options.

Play ball!

Journal: _____

_____

_____

_____

_____

_____

_____

_____

BODY-LIFE NOW!

_____

_____

_____

_____

_____

_____

_____

_____

70. WORKOUT

. . . WORK OUT your own salvation . . . (Philippians 2:12)

———◆———

Everything that you need for ultimate physical development is inside you.

You've already got all the parts . . .

bi's, tri's, lats, delts, pecs, traps, glutes, abs . . .

they're all a part of you *now*.

You just have to work them out to maximize their potential.

Your back is strong –

so are your shoulders and legs.

Don't ignore any parts.

Resist the temptation to only work out your upper body.

You need to be balanced and proportioned and symmetrical,

so make sure that your workout is *total* and *whole*.

In the same way, everything that you need *spiritually* is already inside you.

That's why Paul said to work *OUT* your salvation with fear and trembling.

It all comes from the inside *out* –

the spiritual, as well as the physical.

You must *live* from the inside out . . .

My son, attend to my words; consent and submit to my sayings.

Let them not depart from your sight; keep them in the CENTER of your heart.

For they are life to those who find them, healing and health to all their flesh.

Keep and guard your heart with all vigilance and above all that you guard,

for OUT OF IT FLOW THE SPRINGS OF LIFE. (Proverbs 4:20-23 - AMP)

71.   A PRAYER BEFORE A MORNING WORKOUT

—◆—

Father,

I thank you that this is the day that you have made;

I will rejoice and be glad in it!

Thank you for the gift of life and for a healthy body.

I know that I am fearfully and wonderfully made!

As I work out today, I present my body to you as a living sacrifice.

My body is *your* temple – *your* dwelling place – so I maintain and improve it today as a way to honor *you*.

I call my body well and vital and strong today.

I can do all things through Christ Who strengthens me!

Help me to be led by your Spirit as I workout,

so that I will know how much to *push* myself,

and also when I've done *enough*. Remind me that the fruit of the Spirit is self-control.

Keep me in balance, so that I am able to maintain a proper perspective on the whole process.

And help me to know the difference between feeling good about my body,

and just being conceited and arrogant.

I pray that you keep me safe from injury;

Your angels encamp around me and bear me up in their hands so that I don't

dash my foot against a stone.

Let everything that I do today be for *your* glory.

I am your representative – your ambassador – and I give myself completely to you for your service today.

In Jesus' name, amen.

*Journal:*_____

_____

_____

_____

_____

_____

BODY-LIFE NOW!

_____

_____

_____

_____

_____

_____

_____

72. A PRAYER OF DEDICATION FOR RUNNING A RACE

Father,

Everything that I do is to glorify you,

so I dedicate this (5K, 10K, half marathon, marathon) to your honor.

I will run today and not be weary.

In you I live and MOVE and have my being,

so I celebrate life today by using the body that you have given me for this purpose.

I call my legs strong.

I am strong in the Lord and in the power of His might.

I command my body to line up with your Word, Lord.

I thank you that your angels encamp around me

and keep me from experiencing any injury.

They will keep me from dashing my foot against a stone,

and, therefore, no weapon formed against me during this race can prosper.

I declare the end from the beginning

and say that I *will* finish this race

and will do it in my best possible time.

You, Lord, will be a shade at my right hand,

so that the sun will not smite me by day.

The name of exhaustion, heat stroke, sprained ankle,

shin-splints, or any other negative thing, must bow to the name of Jesus.

I will take dominion in this race today – for your glory.

In Jesus' name, amen.

*Journal:*_____

73.   A PRAYER FOR WEIGHT-LOSS

Father,

I present my body to you as a living sacrifice.

I am not my own; I am bought with a price,

so I take authority over my weight

and I decree that, in my life, the name of gluttony has to bow to the name of Jesus.

The fruit of the Spirit is self-control,

so by the *power* of the Spirit I say that I am disciplined in my diet.

I have the mind of Christ to enable me to make good food choices.

My belly is not my god,

but I seek first the Kingdom of God and His righteousness,

and everything that I need, nutritionally, is added to me.

I will not snare myself by the words of my mouth,

but I will speak about my body in accordance with what I am praying for it.

Help me to choose the workout or exercise that will give me the best results for my body type.

I have a vision for the way that I want my body to be,

and I will not give up on that vision until I realize it.

I *can* be my ideal weight,

because I can do all things through Christ Who strengthens me.

My weight does not control me – *I* control my weight!

You have set before me life and death, and I choose life!

In Jesus' name, amen.

*Journal:*_____

_____

_____

_____

_____

_____

_____

_____

BODY-LIFE NOW!

_____

_____

_____

_____

_____

_____

_____

74.   A CONFESSION OF HEALTH AND HEALING

In Jesus' name, I call my body *healed* and *whole*.

By His stripes I am healed!

My health springs forth, speedily.

The same Spirit that raised Jesus from the dead dwells in me, and quickens my mortal body.

Jehovah Rapha takes sickness away from my midst

and, because I am Abraham's seed, none of the plagues of the Egyptians can come upon me.

The name of my every sickness, disease or pain has to bow to the name of Jesus.

I command every cell of my body to come under His authority

and to line up with His Word.

I am not afraid of symptoms of sickness, because God has not given me a spirit of fear,

but of power, and of love, and of a sound mind.

My faith makes me whole. My faith is the evidence of things not seen.

Bless the Lord, O my soul, and *all* that is within me bless His holy name!

Bless the Lord, and forget not all His benefits,

Who forgives all of my iniquities,

and heals *all* of my diseases.

Lord, put a watch over my mouth, so that my words are words of *health* and *life*.

Death and life are in the power of *my* tongue.

You are the God who heals me . . .

"The Lord, my Healer" is your name.

Today, I boldly and confidently say, "IT IS WELL!"

*Journal:*_____

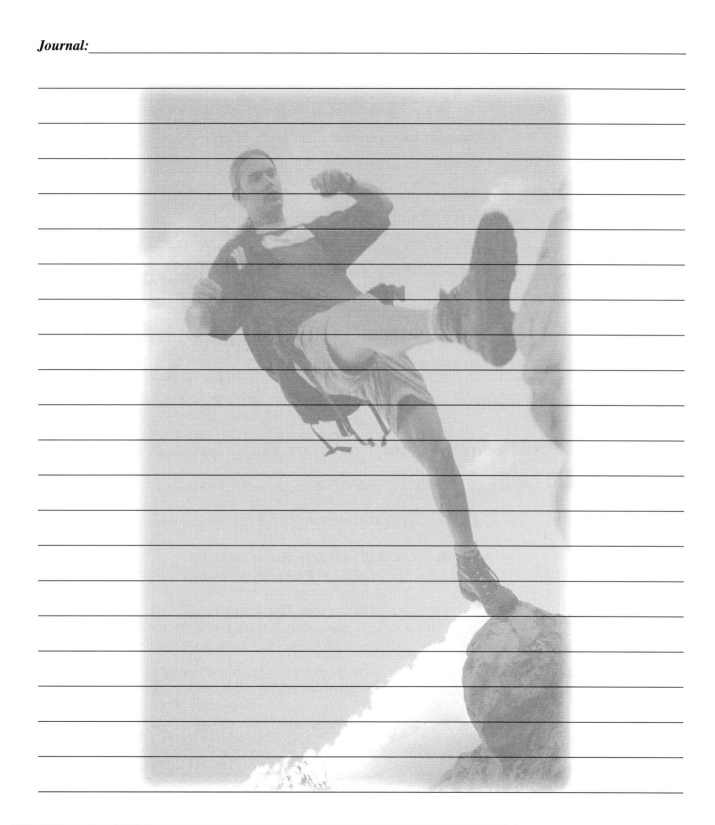

75. PROMISES FOR A LONG LIFE

———◆———

Many people who do not know how to rightly divide the Word of God take Psalm 90:10 out of context and use it to limit man's lifespan to 70 to 80 years. But this verse refers to the length of life of those who wandered in the wilderness in the time of Moses, which was shortened so that the old generation could die off within the 40 years. The days of these 40 years could actually be numbered (v.12). Ordinarily, days cannot be numbered, because we are not living through a special curse, as was Israel in the wilderness (Numbers 14:29-36). No authority is given here for setting the length of a person's life at *"threescore and ten."* Some men lived much longer, even when Moses wrote this, and many have lived longer in *every* generation. If there *is* any God-decreed limit to lifespan, it is found in Genesis 6:3:

> *Then God said, "I'm not going to breathe life into men and women endlessly.*
> *Eventually they're going to die; FROM NOW ON THEY CAN*
> *EXPECT A LIFE SPAN OF 120 YEARS."*

Besides taking care of your body, here are the promises that you can claim to prolong your life:

> *Good friend, don't forget all I've taught you; take to heart my commands.*
> *They'll help you LIVE A LONG, LONG TIME, a LONG LIFE lived full and well. (Proverbs 3:1,2)*

> *With one hand she [wisdom] gives LONG LIFE, with the other she confers recognition. (Proverbs 3:16)*

> *Dear friend, take my advice; it will ADD YEARS TO YOUR LIFE. (Proverbs 4:10)*

> *For by me [Wisdom from God] your days shall be multiplied,*
> *and the YEARS OF YOUR LIFE SHALL BE INCREASED. (Proverbs 9:11- AMP)*

> *Children, do what your parents tell you. This is only right.*
> *"Honor your father and mother" is the first commandment that has a promise attached to it,*
> *namely, "so you will live well and have a LONG LIFE." (Ephesians 6:1-3)*

> *It is appointed for men to die once (Hebrews 9:27)*, but, as you can see from the Scriptures,
> *you* have as much or more say in *when that time is going to be,* as God does!

Live long and prosper!

---

*Journal:*_____

BODY-LIFE NOW!

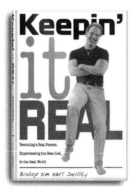

Keepin' It Real

Becoming a Real Person,
Experiencing the Real God,
in the Real World

You've never read a book quite like *Keepin' It Real!* In its pages, Bishop Swilley candidly examines an unusually wide array of subjects . . . the reality TV phenomenon . . . pop culture . . . history . . . politics . . . self-esteem . . . prosperity . . . success . . . parenting . . . multiculturalism . . . New Age philosophy . . . world religions . . . political correctness . . . racism . . . sexism . . . tolerance . . . activism . . . technology . . . addiction . . . eschatology . . . dispensationalism . . . the antichrist . . . orthodoxy . . . prayer . . . the Holy Spirit . . . destiny . . . purpose . . . vision . . . and much more . . . and addresses how they all relate to the Kingdom of God in the now!

But *Keepin' it Real* is also about *you* and how you can develop the courage and confidence to be yourself at all times and to live your *real* life without compromise. Socially relevant, thought-provoking, and theologically edgy, *Keepin' it Real* is a modern manifesto for REAL PEOPLE EXPERIENCING THE REAL GOD IN THE REAL WORLD.®

If you're ready to get *real*, get this book!

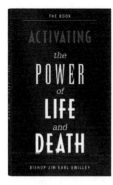

Activating the Power of Life and Death

It's Your Life . . .
It's Your Choice . . .
YOU CHOOSE!

God has given you the power to choose life or death, blessing or cursing. By the words of your mouth, you determine the quality of your life. This powerful book will help put you in charge of your life and future.

A Year In The Now!

a dynamic devotional dedicated to
the daily discovery of destiny.

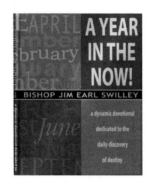

Would you like to . . .

. . . discover your destiny?
. . . perceive your purpose?
. . . validate your vision?
. . . reinforce your relationships?
. . . strengthen your self-esteem?
. . . overcome your obstacles?
. . . feed your faith?

You can . . . this year!
You can . . . by living in the now!
You can . . . one day at a time!

God is on your side! He is available to assist you in the pursuit of your potential as you develop the diligence to seriously search out your personal path for growth into greatness! Through seeking first His Kingdom and righteousness, you can become the person that He created you to be!

You can ONLY find God's Kingdom in the eternal "NOW" as you endeavor to experience Him in your everyday existence. Kingdom-seeking consists of a constant effort to embrace the now and a commitment to the continual conforming of your consciousness to it. This empowers and enables you to escape the mental distractions produced by living in the past or in the future, so that you can comprehend a real Christ for your current real circumstances!

A YEAR IN THE NOW! is a devotional designed to deliver a doable format for the daily development of your eternal life – to help you think creatively, beyond your familiar, time-bound comfort zones. These positive and powerful affirmations will provide the help you need to progressively put your life on the right track in realistic increments. You don't have to become overwhelmed by the tremendous task of trying to lead a "now life" in a "yesterday/tomorrow world." You can do it day by day!

This is your year to change your world! You can change your world by changing your mind! You can change your mind one day at a time!

It's time for a fresh start, and you can start right NOW!

What others have to say about *A Year In The Now!* . . .

When my dear friend, Bishop Jim Swilley sent me a copy of his new daily devotional, *A Year In The Now!*, I stopped everything I was doing and couldn't put it down . . . that is until my wife took it out of my hands and I have had to pry it back from her ever since. Jim is one of the most effective, prolific, and unique communicators I have ever met. He breaks down deep and profound truth and makes it palatable for all of us in such a practical way that just reading the principles and reciting the affirmations increases our life skills. The days are broken down into seven key principles a day, seven being the number of alignment between heaven and earth (4 being the number of earth, and three of heaven), whereby applying the seven daily truths your heart and mind are aligned with heaven's best and you are automatically brought into the kind of agreement that gets results in your life. If you want to get the "more" out of your daily life that has been promised to you in Christ I want to encourage you to get your hands on *A Year In The Now!* and make it a part of your daily spiritual discipline and focus. Oh yea, and if anyone else gets their hands on your copy in your family . . . buy another one because you won't get it back quick enough!

Dr. Mark J. Chironna
The Master's Touch International Church
Orlando, Florida

Your devotional, *A Year in the Now!*, reads as a personal message to me. Each day I am encouraged - God is doing a new thing in the NOW! This devotional reinforces that God is working His plan in all things that affect my family and ministry. My destiny continues to unfold so that others will see my good works and glorify the Father.

Germaine Copeland
Author of Prayers That Avail Much Family Books

Deeply profound, yet 'DO-ably' practical. That's how I describe Bishop Jim Earl Swilley's *A Year In The Now!* daily devotional. Bishop Jim's 'easy to read' style of communication, combined with his witty grouping together of words that start with the same letter, define this devotional as a delightful way to delve deeper into your divine destiny as a daily discipline. Profound and practical, it's the perfect proponent to promote your personal progress.

Doug Fortune
Trumpet Call Ministry

A Year In The Now! by Bishop Jim Earl Swilley, is extraordinary and powerful, giving day by day guidance on how to be strong in the Lord through seven pearls of wisdom each day. Seven! This is God's number for completeness and fulfillment. Through A Year In The Now!, God is truly using Bishop Swilley in a mighty way to unlock the wonderful mystery of the gospel so that each of us can live abundantly, and serve God abundantly, in the now!

David Scott
United States Congressman, Georgia

To receive a full listing of Bishop Swilley's products, write or call:

Jim Earl Swilley Ministries
P.O. Box 80876
Conyers, GA 30013

Phone: 678-607-3113
Fax: 770-922-5337
E-mail: products@churchinthenow.org
Internet: www.churchinthenow.org